Personal Fitness Training

Beyond The Basics

Joe Cannon, MS

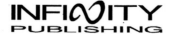
INFINITY
PUBLISHING

ISBN 0-7414-4984-6

Joe Cannon's Website: www.Joe-Cannon.com

Published by:

INFINITY
PUBLISHING

1094 New DeHaven Street, Suite 100
West Conshohocken, PA 19428-2713
Info@buybooksontheweb.com
www.buybooksontheweb.com
Toll-free (877) BUY BOOK
Local Phone (610) 941-9999
Fax (610) 941-9959

Printed in the United States of America

Published August 2010

TABLE of CONTENTS

For Margaret Lynch Cannon, my 104 year old
grandmother and oldest personal training "client".
It was a pleasure.

Acknowledgments

No book is the work of only a single person but rather is the collaboration of many others who worked behind the scenes, some without even knowing it. Let me take a moment to thank some of those people now.

As always, much thanks also to Kelly Bixler my proofreader and niece. It's good to have someone in the family to catch all my typos.

This text would be a lot different if it were not for the efforts of Marcie Parke, the official illustrator of this book. Thanks for your hard word and dedication.

Thanks to my buddies, Chris Blessing, Paul Coppola, Tim DiFelice, Adam Freedman and Bill Leinhauser for their friendship over the years and for helping me in their own unique ways.

Lastly, thanks to all of the fitness trainers who urged me to write this book. Your questions, emails over the years and comments were instrumental in my writing a more user-friendly book that I could have alone. Thank you all very much!

Start Reading Here

Congratulations! You are holding what I believe to be one of the most user-friendly books on personal fitness training in the world today. Within these pages, is the book I've wanted to write for a very long time; a book that gives you the "big picture" of personal training, providing you with not only the science stuff that fitness trainers need to know but also the *art* of how to apply that science to the real world. I'll endeavor to do this by basically trying to have a conversation with you as if I were sitting right next to you, sharing with you my own voyage of discovery; the facts I've learned over the years as well as personal stories and even mistakes that I've made along the way.

Based on my own experiences, I have condensed some of the science concepts, to what I felt was most useful to fitness trainers and, where possible, place that science within the context of fitness and health to help foster learning and hopefully spark your imagination.

Fitness professionals are primarily educators and often find themselves on the front lines fielding many questions. Because of this, I've purposely tried answer some of those questions that I know you will one day be asked– and hopefully questions you may have asked yourself from time to time.

No matter whether you are just starting out as a personal trainer or have been in the field for many years, it is my sincere hope that what I have created here will be of some help to you as you pursue your passion and help others achieve their dreams…

Joe Cannon

Let's Roll!

Chapter 1

BECOMING A PERSONAL TRAINER

There is a good chance that if you are reading these words you are either thinking about becoming a personal fitness trainer or you are already one and are looking for additional information. In either case, this chapter is good to read because it will explain a lot about what it means to be a personal trainer as well as give helpful information whether, you are a veteran or just starting out in the industry.

What is a Personal Fitness Trainer?

Some may think the answer to this is a no-brainer but I think it deserves mention. A personal trainer is a health and fitness professional who is usually contracted to perform private or semi-private exercise sessions with a person or small group of people. Notice the word *professional* in that definition. Personal trainers are professionals just like accountants, lawyers, business people, etc. Personal trainers are also members of the healthcare system as are physicians, nurses, physical therapists, pharmacists, chiropractors, massage therapists and occupational therapists to name a few. While these professionals have skills and expertise that personal trainers may not have, it is also true that personal trainers have knowledge and proficiency in areas that these other professionals may not possess. Because of their connection to health, personal trainers should be familiar with how exercise impacts health. They should also be familiar with various principles of exercise science and how to apply those principles.

As professionals, personal trainers should strive to conduct themselves in a professional manner when they are in public or with clients. Several easy ways to do this include:

1. **Dressing appropriately.** If you are employed at a health club, adhere to its dress code. Maintaining proper attire helps members know who you are and avoids confusion. Baggy clothes are usually not appropriate as they may get caught in equipment. Perfume and cologne should be modest if worn at all. Some people may be allergic to overly powerful cologne or perfume. In addition, if you are working with asthmatics, wear no scents at all as it may exacerbate their condition. For those who are self employed, dress modestly. Probably the best and most functional outfits might be khakis, a collared shirt and sneakers.

2. **Using business cards.** Business cards are one of the easiest ways you have to advertise yourself and your services as well as tell the world that you have your act together.

3. **Being a people person.** You have to like helping people to be fitness professional. You can have all the knowledge in the world, but if you can't talk to others in a way that makes them feel comfortable, that's a problem.

4. **Maintaining a professional relationship with clients.** Yes, of course you are going to find some clients that you are going to count among your friends. That's normal. Just be sure if you are working with a client in the capacity of a personal trainer that you do not cross the line.

Intervening in marital disagreements would be an example of this. It goes without saying – but I will say it anyway – personal trainers do not have inappropriate relations (that means sex!) with clients! As a personal trainer, you represent an entire industry of tens of thousands of people and what you do reflects upon everyone else in the industry. Aside from embarrassment for all parties, serious violations of professional conduct can also result in the revoking of your fitness certification. If you are serious about being a fitness professional and passionate about your trade then there is a good chance that you may go from relative obscurity to being well known. You don't want anybody who can drag skeletons out of your closet and fizzle out your rising star.

5. **Maintaining a network of other health professionals.** No personal trainer knows everything or can be all things to all people. To give people the best possible service, all personal trainers should have contacts of other health care professionals when their client's needs fall outside the scope of a personal trainer's practice. Registered dietitians, physical therapists, occupational therapists, massage therapists, and chiropractors are all good examples.

6. **Keeping personal info private.** Because personal training is personal, you will likely be privy to an assortment of personal information about your clients. Some information they may tell you in confidence and other things you may just overhear in passing. It is important that all of this information stay in your "lockbox". Divulging personal information is the fastest way to lose a client and give you a bad reputation.

7. **Staying educated.** People are pretty smart and as a fitness professional, you are going to be asked all sorts of questions. Obviously you can't know everything but the best way to be prepared is to keep up with what's going on in your field. Reading books, attending seminars, watching DVDs, and subscribing to trade journals are some of the easiest ways to stay on top of things.

PT or CPT?

Some personal trainers refer to themselves (and what they do) as "PTs". This makes sense since the two first letters in *personal training* are PT. That being said, the letters PT are usually understood by the public to mean physical therapy. So, to avoid confusion, the acronym CPT, for "certified personal trainer" was devised. Some personal trainers even have the letters CPT behind their names and on their business cards. When in doubt it's probably wise not to list what you do as "PT" as it may annoy physical therapists who had the moniker first.

Where Do Personal Trainers Work and How Much Do They Make?

According to the US Bureau of Labor and Statistics, there are over 60,000 certified personal trainers in America.[40] The actual number of personal trainers may be much higher than this given that some may not be certified. Personal trainers are employed in a number of fields with the majority being employed in fitness centers and health clubs. Salaries for personal trainers can vary with location as well as education and experience but according to the US Bureau of Labor and Statistics, the average annual income for trainers in 2004 was about $25,000.[40] While that may not seem like much, the top

10% of personal trainers in America earned over $55,000.[40] For trainers who listed themselves as self employed, average annual income was higher yet.[40] It is interesting to note that the field of personal fitness training is expected to be one of the fastest growing industries through the year 2014.[40]

What's Better: A Degree or Certification?

For those just starting (and those who have been in the field for a while) the question often arises as to which is better: a college degree or fitness certification? Some personal trainers do indeed have college degrees and this may appeal to some employers and clients. However, a college degree does not necessarily mean that you know personal training. It is a fact that many college exercise degree programs either do not teach or spend very little time discussing the *art* of personal training. For this reason many employers also recommend that their personal trainers have fitness certifications as well.

Today there are hundreds of fitness certifications to choose from. Some of the larger and more recognized organizations include the American Aerobics Association International/ International Sports Medication Association (AAAI/ISMA), Aerobics and Fitness Association of America (AFAA), American College of Sports Medicine (ACSM), American Council on Exercise (ACE), International Sports Sciences Association (ISSA), National Academy of Sports Medicine (NASM) and National Strength and Conditioning Association (NSCA).

While all certifying organizations essentially teach similar topics, they may differ in the time they spend on subjects and the importance that different topics rank on their certification exams. Also, some certifications may require a college degree before you are allowed to take the exam. Many also require you to have a current CPR and/or AED certification as well.

Most organizations also offer several different certifications. For example, many organizations offer certifications that deal with sports nutrition, weight management, aerobics and working with special needs individuals. In addition, certifications also differ in cost.

Obtaining a CPR Certification

In addition to a fitness certification, it is wise to also have a CPR certification as well. Obtaining this cert *before* you sign up for a fitness certification is a good idea because many organizations may require this as a prerequisite for taking their test. Also, many health clubs will require a current CPR certification prior to employment. CPR certifications are relatively inexpensive, costing around $50 in some areas. Both the American Red Cross (www.redcross.org) and American Heart Association (www.americanheart.org) websites let you connect with certifications in your area. CPR classes are also offered at local colleges, hospitals, YMCAs and fire stations.

In addition to CPR, it may be wise to also obtain an AED certification. AED stands for automated external defibrillator. This is a portable device which, in the event of a heart attack, can help keep a person alive until help arrives. Many health clubs now have AEDs on site and require staff and managers to be properly trained in its use. To obtain proper training in the use of an AED, contact either the Red Cross or American Heart Association websites.

What's the Best Certification?

People often wonder which is the best fitness certification. Honestly, the lay public usually doesn't know one cert from another. Also some certifications, while very good, may assume the student has advanced knowledge prior to taking a certification exam or discuss topics in language that only Albert Einstein could understand. I personally have textbooks that I have to read a few times before

I know what the author is talking about! The bottom line is to not get hung up on which is the best cert. The trick is to find a certification that's reputable, teaches you what you need to know to work safely with others, allows you to get re-certified relatively easily and, in my opinion, is cost effective for your budget. Whichever certification you obtain, the most important thing you can do is to continue to educate yourself. A certification, by itself, only demonstrates you know *minimum* requirements. A certification does not mean you know everything. You wouldn't want a doctor who only knew the minimum, would you? Of course you wouldn't. The same goes for your clients. Having a certification plus six-pack abs may get you a few clients but if you can't accurately answer a question like "why does my urine look like coke-a-cola after I work out," you are at a big disadvantage and you probably won't keep those clients long. *Knowledge is power* and is more valuable to people then the size of ones biceps. Consumers are very smart these days and they look for professionals who can save them time not only working out but also as they search for answers regarding their health.

Chapter 2

WHAT TO DO WHEN YOU GET A NEW CLIENT

For those just starting out in the business, one of the most frequently asked questions is "what do I do when I get a new client?" This makes perfect sense given that many certifications and college degree programs tend to focus only on the nuts-and-bolts science of personal training. While personal training is very science based, the rubber meets the road stuff of the profession should not take a back seat. Both are closely intertwined. All the knowledge in the world won't help if you can't obtain a client and foster a working relationship. Because of this, let's now review some of the steps that you should be taking when you get that client – whether it's your very first personal training client, or your 100th.

The Initial Interview

The initial interview is the first meeting that you will have with a new client. This time can be used to gather valuable information as well as to demonstrate to the new client your professionalism. Unless the client specifically asks you to call them by their first name, addressing them in the formal manner is always preferable. Whenever possible, the initial interview should be conducted in a private area, such as an office. This is because the client will be divulging private, sensitive information. In addition, conducting the interview in private can also help reduce uneasiness that the client may feel during any fitness testing that occurs. Taking circumference or body fat measurements in a public area is one of the fastest ways to make a new client feel uneasy. While this may not be an issue for fitness trainers who travel to people's homes, for gyms and health clubs that have limited space, this can be a difficult obstacle to overcome.

Another advantage of the initial interview is that it provides a time for the trainer and client to get to know each other and engage in conversation. While on the surface, this may seem secondary to the main goals of the interview, this can help you gather valuable information. For example, it is sometimes said that over 80% of a spoken sentence is nonverbal (i.e., body language). Nonverbal cues like poor posture, not making eye contact, folding of arms, etc. can provide valuable information. For example, someone who timidly sits in a chair and doesn't remove his/her coat indoors may be signs that the person is depressed or nervous. The ability to recognize nonverbal signs can be an invaluable tool that many pay little attention to.

During the initial interview (if not before), fitness professionals should provide their personal contact information such as cell phone number and/or email address. Providing this information can help the client schedule sessions as well cancel sessions if an emergency arises. All personal trainers should provide this service to their clients. Just about any home computer can easily make business cards and business card paper can be cheaply purchased from any office supply store. Ideally, only one phone number should be given: the phone number you are most likely to answer. Providing several phone numbers increases the chances of a missed call and increases the likelihood that you will miss an appointment. Also, the phone number given should have voicemail so clients can leave a message if you are not able to answer. Your personal voicemail greeting should be professional sounding and easy to understand. Likewise, it is in the trainer's best interest to provide a *professional*, easy to spell email address. For example, "yourname@gmail.com". Email addresses that are lewd or suggestive are inappropriate for business purposes and are one of the fastest ways to make a bad impression on a new client.

The Health History Form

A man joins a health club and hires a personal trainer to help him get back in shape. After about 10 minutes into their first workout, the man starts to look tired and has to sit down. The trainer becomes concerned and asks if the man is ok to which the man replies *I'll be ok in a few minutes; I had open heart surgery three weeks ago and I'm still recovering!* Now, can you imagine the shock on the face of the personal trainer who, until that very moment, had no idea that the man had undergone such a major surgical procedure! This is actually a true story that was told to me by the personal trainer himself! I mention this because it highlights one of my "rules of personal training" which is: *Never work with someone until you know his/her personal health history.*

The fact cannot be stated enough that personal trainers MUST know who they are dealing with. Don't assume that people are healthy because they are in a health club or "look" fit. A topic that is not often talked about is that ticking time bombs walk the floors of every health club in the world. I say this not to frighten you but to arm you with the knowledge that this is so. Now that you know this, you are already better prepared if (and when) you encounter one of these individuals. So, how can you identify high risk people? Have them complete a health history questionnaire. All health history forms will probably have the same major sections. They include: personal contact information, personal and family health history, medication usage and even fitness history.

Personal Contact Information

This section of a health history form includes data such as name, address, phone number, email address as well as the name/phone number of the primary care physician and emergency contact information. It is very important that all personal and medical history data be kept private. Also, fitness professionals should refrain from discussing a client's personal or private information with other colleagues in a way that would allow for the client to be identified. In addition, the client's specific conditions, etc., should not be discussed in public settings like restaurants. Personal trainers should keep all of their clients' information in an organized filing system such as in a filing cabinet that has the ability to be locked. This is especially important for hospital-based fitness centers that may be subject to special privacy regulations.

Personal Health History

This section is where you collect information on the client's current and past health status. It is here that questions pertaining medical conditions and injuries are asked. Other questions can include those pertaining to cholesterol levels, blood pressure and cigarette smoking habits.

Fitness professionals, who encounter clients with serious medical issues like heart disease, diabetes, etc., should refer them to the client's primary care physician and obtain a written approval note from that physician before exercise training begins. This serves not only as an extra measure of safety for the individual but also may help the fitness professional down the road in the event of litigation. Obtaining a note from a qualified medical professional can also been viewed as a marketing opportunity for personal trainers. As many know, it can be difficult to schedule a meeting with a physician because they are busy with patients, paperwork, and other tasks that make demands on their time. By referring high risk people back to their physician prior to training, you open up an opportunity for the physician to get to know you better. More importantly, doing so also demonstrates to the physician your level of competency and the care you provide for their patients.

Family Health History

Several years ago, I was told by the management of the health club where I worked at that they would no longer need me to work on the weekends because the club wasn't very busy during those times. I felt that it was a mistake not to have any fitness staff on duty, but for reasons only management can answer, the club stuck to its guns. Unfortunately, one weekend, about a month later everyone's worst nightmare came true when a man, in his mid-30s died while working out. Now, while you might automatically think that's the end of the story, it's not. You see, I later learned that the man had a brother who, just a few years before, also died. I tell you this story to emphasize the importance of knowing the health history of a client's immediate family members. In general, those whose mother, aunt or sister died suddenly or had a heart attack before the age of 65 or whose father, uncle or brother passed away or had a heart attack before the age of 55, may be at an increased risk of early death from heart disease.[1] These people should be referred to their physician prior to training. In addition, knowledge of family health issues may enable the trainer to help his/her client more fully. For example, if a family history of osteoporosis is known it may be possible, through proper exercise, to reduce its occurrence in the client in the future.

Heart Disease Risk Factors[1]

Risk Factor	Specific Information
Family History	Heart attack, heart disease surgery or sudden death before the age of 55 in father or immediate relative (son, brother) or before the age of 65 in mother or other immediate relative (sister, daughter)
Cigarette Smoking	Someone who is a current smoker or one who quit smoking in the last 6 months
High Blood Pressure	Blood pressure greater than 140/90 mm Hg or someone on medications for high blood pressure
High Cholesterol Levels	Total cholesterol greater than 200 mg/dl or HDL less than 40 mg /dl or someone taking medications for high cholesterol. Also someone whose LDL cholesterol is greater than 100 mg/dl
Obesity	Having a BMI greater than 30 kg/m^2 or having a waist circumference greater than 100 cm
Non-Active Lifestyle	Those not regularly engaging at least 30 minutes of sustained activity most days of the week

Note: an HDL of 60 mg/dl or better is considered a "negative risk factor" for heart disease. In other words, this lowers the chance that heart disease develops.[1] Aerobic exercise does a good job at raising HDL.

Who is Low Risk and Who is High Risk?

By using the preceding table of heart disease risk factors it is possible to estimate a person's risk of heart disease.[1]

Low Risk	Children, adolescents, men younger than 45 and women younger than 55 who have no symptoms of heart disease and have no more than 1 risk factor
Moderate Risk	Men 45 or older and women 55 or older or those who have 2 or more risk factors
High Risk	Person's who have heart disease, diabetes or lung disease or those who have one or more heart disease signs or symptoms

Medication Use

Fitness professionals are generally not physicians or pharmacists and are not expected to understand how medications work. That being said, it's a good idea to inquire about the types of medications people are taking because it can help you help them better. For example, some medications (e.g., beta blockers) can affect the degree to which people can exercise. This is important information to know about when designing an exercise program. When discussing medications, the goal should be viewed as another opportunity to identify people who are high risk. When you encounter people who are taking medications to treat serious conditions like high blood pressure, diabetes, heart disease, kidney disorders, cancer, etc., they should be referred back to their physician and instructed to obtain a written note from their doctor stating that they are medically cleared to exercise. The note should be kept for safekeeping in the person's file. Personal trainers, like all fitness professionals, are members of the healthcare continuum. That spectrum of diverse medical and health care practitioners works best when the client's primary care physician is kept in the loop with what his/her patient is doing. Exercise can definitely help; however some people should get medical clearance before they begin an exercise program.

Conditions That Require a Physician's Approval*

Heart disease	Chest pain at rest	Emphysema
High blood pressure	Chest pain during exercise	Pregnancy
Kidney disorders	Diabetes	Cancer
Prior heart attack	HIV/AIDS	Asthma
Pacemaker	Morbid Obesity	Sedentary lifestyle
Heart surgery	Early death of parents	Stroke

* This is a partial list

Related to medications, some trainers may also inquire about the use of dietary supplements. Studies show that most Americans take supplements ranging from something as simple as a multivitamin to exotic herbs, minerals and other products reputed to help any number of conditions. For the record, there are good supplements and those that are not so good. The trick is figuring out which is which. It's a fact, many supplements can interact with medical issues and medications. Just because a supplement can be sold over the counter does not mean it has no side effects. Because of this I highly recommend my book, *Nutritional Supplements: What Works and Why*, which reviews supplement side effects that most people in fitness have never heard of. That book can be obtained on my website www.Joe-Cannon.com.

Fitness History

Obviously, it's a good idea to know about the past (and present) experiences your client has had with exercise. Questions for this section can include:

> - What types of physical activities do you enjoy?
> - What physical activities have you done in the past?
> - Do you participate in any sports?
> - Do you have difficulty performing any physical activity?

Questions like these help tease out information about a person's likes and dislikes and can assist with designing an effective exercise program that is not only enjoyable but also addresses any specific needs the person may have. For example, people indicating that they play a particular sport or activity provide an opportunity to incorporate movements that can help strengthen muscles to help them play their sport better as well as reduce the risk of injury.

The PAR-Q

Besides the health history form, one may also wish to administer a separate document called the PAR-Q. PAR-Q stands for *Physical Activity Readiness Questionnaire*. Basically, the PAR-Q is a one page form that can help identify people who may not be suitable for exercise. The PAR Q is appropriate for people 15-69 years of age. This form is the very *minimum* that should be completed prior to working with someone.[1] The PAR-Q, though, is not foolproof and in reality should be part of a comprehensive screening process that includes a health history form. The PAR-Q consists of a short series of easy to understand questions. Bottom Line: if the person answers *yes* to any of the questions, there is a possibility that he/she may have significant medical issues and should see their doctor first before starting an exercise program.

PAR-Q Questions[1]

---

1. Has your doctor ever said that you have a heart condition and that you should only do physical activity recommended by a doctor?
2. Do you feel pain in your chest when you do physical activity?
3. In the past month, have you had chest pain when you were not doing physical activity?
4. Do you lose your balance because of dizziness or do you ever lose consciousness?
5. Do you have a bone or joint problem that could be made worse by a change in your physical activity?
6. Is your doctor currently prescribing drugs (for example, water pills) for your blood pressure or heart condition?
7. Do you know of any other reason why you should not do physical activity?

The actual PAR-Q form can be viewed online by connecting to an Internet search engine and typing in the phrase "PAR-Q and You." Aside from its use by fitness professionals, fitness centers may also use this document. In other words, if all new health club members completed the PAR-Q prior to joining a health club, it might help decrease the number of high-risk people who joined without their doctor's approval.

Additional Forms

The Waiver

Before the first training session occurs, all clients should complete a legally binding waiver of liability. This is also sometimes called a Release form. This form can help protect the fitness professional if something unfortunate occurs during training. Having a properly worded waiver can help reduce a successful lawsuit from occurring. Most fitness centers have carefully worded waivers that all members sign prior to joining. Some fitness centers may also have additional *personal trainer waivers* that people sign prior to working with a personal trainer. If you are working in a health club, ask the manager or owner about their specific guidelines regarding waivers. Self-employed personal trainers must have their own waiver. Regardless of where you work—self employed or at a health club—waivers, like all client information, should be kept in a safe place.

Ideally, the waiver should be drawn up by an attorney in your state who has knowledge of Contract Law and the health and fitness industry. When searching for a lawyer you may want to ask them if they have written documents like waivers for fitness professionals in the past.

The sizes of the words on some waivers I have seen are so small that people may have difficulty reading them. Thus, the font size should be legible. You may want to have both hard copies (paper copies) as well as copies stored on your computer as a pdf file. That way you can fax or email copies to clients if you need to. Your attorney can help you with this.

In addition, it is important that the fitness professional explain the nature of the waiver to the client. People must understand what the document means. When discussing the waiver do not downplay its significance. In other words don't say "This is something that I have to do; it really doesn't mean much". By signing the waiver, the client is essentially waiving many (but not all) of their rights to take legal action. This is very significant! Downplaying the significance of the waiver might open up a legal loophole that could come back to bite you in the event you ever go to court. An attorney can also advise you on the best way to explain the waiver to people. Also, keep in mind that waivers may not protect you in all circumstances. For example, waivers may not protect you if you perform tasks that fall outside you role as a personal trainer (e.g., diagnosing medical problems).

Lastly, keep in mind laws vary from state to state. A waiver created for a fitness center or personal trainer in Texas may not hold up if you're working in Massachusetts. Thus, it is not a good idea for trainers to copy a waiver used by someone else or one found on the Internet. The bottom line is that you really do need to get an attorney. Fitness trainers are usually not lawyers and are not expected to be. Save yourself the headache of trying to figure this stuff out on your own. An attorney can help save you a lot of time and legal fees down the road.

Liability Insurance

Just as you probably have insurance for your home, car, and health, personal trainers should also have liability insurance. While personal trainers who work at health clubs may be covered by the club's policy (check to make sure), self-employed personal trainers MUST have their own liability insurance.

While not the norm, some health clubs may allow outside trainers (who are not employees) to work with clients at their facility. In this instance, the club will require you to provide not only your fitness and CPR certifications but also proof of liability insurance as well. The same is true for trainers who work with clients at fitness centers that are associated with the client's condominium or apartment complex.

Many companies exist that can provide liability insurance. Also, the organization by which you are certified can often point you in the right direction. Prices usually range from $200-$500 per year. Keep in mind that liability insurance may not cover you for everything.

Trainer/Client Agreement

The agreement between the client and the trainer is a document that is sometimes used to help outline the responsibilities of both parties. It may not be legally binding; however, the client and trainer both normally sign the form. This is usually done because people tend to be more likely to follow through with something if they sign their name to it. This form contains information regarding dressing properly for workouts, showing up on time for workouts, giving a reasonable amount of notice (that you specify) if they (or the trainer) must cancel a workout and so on.

Goals Sheet

Obviously the fitness professional should know the reasons why the client has sought out his/her help. This is where the goals sheet comes in handy. Unfortunately, it has been my personal observation that many trainers miss the power of learning about goals. This is probably because, as many fitness professionals will tell you, most people have the same goals – tone up, lose weight, etc. After seeing the same goals day after day, month after month, it's likely that trainers may take them for granted. That being said, I'd like to suggest a new way to gather information on goals. Have all clients write a paragraph for each goal they have. Ask them to list all the reasons why they want to attain their goal. Advise them to be as specific and honest as possible. You might assign this as homework since it will take them some time. Reassure them that nobody will ever view what they have written and that their information will be kept confidential. This is crucial because what they will probably write will be their private, innermost thoughts and feelings. Having people commit to writing their goals in this way helps them take ownership of those goals. In essence, they have taken a small step. By committing to a small step like this, they are more likely to take the bigger step of achieving their goals. If they list more than one goal, ask them to prioritize them. For example, put a "1" next to the goal that's most important and so on.

When you have their written goals, review them with the client on a regular basis (e.g., once a week). This should be done in private. Ask them what they feel have been their triumphs during the previous week (this helps reinforce good behavior) and what have been their setbacks. Write everything down and store the information in their file, which should be kept in a locked area like a file cabinet. When dealing with setbacks, try to design strategies to avoid or better deal with problem areas in the future.

Nutrition Assessment

Some fitness professionals also include a sheet on which clients can list the types of foods they eat. This is sometimes called a 3-day food journal (some use a week-long food journal). Some fitness centers may use this as an opportunity to introduce members to other services they offer, like nutritional counseling or special educational programs geared toward weight loss. Whatever the reason, if you have clients complete a food journal, make sure they only list foods eaten during "typical" days. Foods eaten on special events, like weddings, etc. should not be listed. For more information on nutrition and sports nutrition, read my book, *Nutrition Essentials*, available at www.Joe-Cannon.com.

Summary: Getting Off to a Good Start with New Clients

1. Arrive early for appointments
2. Listen to clients needs/concerns
3. Have all relevant forms handy and ready for client
4. Provide your contact information
5. Be professional

After the First Meeting: What's Next?

Now that you've met with your client and he or she has completed all of the necessary paperwork. What's next? Let's assume that you both have agreed to meet three times a week. After you agree to meet at a specified time, arrive for the session at least 10 minutes early if you work in a health club. That way, you have a little time to get everything you need before the session begins. If you are a fitness trainer who goes to people's homes/offices, arrive on time for the session if not a few minutes early. If you are going to people's homes or offices, odds are they are doing stuff before you arrive so if you get to them too soon, it may complicate their daily schedule. Usually five minutes prior to the session is ok. If you are going to be late for a session, call the client and inform them. If you work at a health club call the front desk and have them notify the client when he/she arrives (add the club's number in your cell phone to make it easier). When you meet the client, shake his/her hand and address the person in a formal manner (Mr. or Mrs. for example).

You should be appropriately dressed for the session. That means wearing the club's uniform or if you're a self employed trainer, wearing something casual yet professional like a warm up suit, etc. Breath mints or gum may also be something to consider (remember, personal training is personal!). Clothes that emulate the latest urban/hip hop fashion trends are usually not appropriate. Think about it. If you're training a 50-year old businessman, will he be able to identify with a trainer who looks like he/she walked out of a music video? Probably not. In fact, that man probably wouldn't hire that trainer. In personal training, appearances do matter to a degree. True, they are not the main factor but when it comes to first impressions, people unfortunately do tend to judge a person by the clothes he/she wears.

Let's assume you've already developed the exercise program for your client and are taking him/her through it. Before the workout begins it's always a good idea to ask the person how he/she is feeling. I usually make it a point to ask people if they have any pains, especially in the neck, shoulders, elbows, low back, knees or ankles. By asking them this, it is my hope to remind them of any other issues, injuries or problems that they should communicate to me before the workout begins. I do this for all clients, whether I see them infrequently or several times a week.

All workouts should have a warm-up period of 5-10 minutes to help prepare the body for exercise. You can be present during the warm-up or advise the client to perform it him/herself. For people with special needs, it's a good idea if you are present for the warm-up, for safety reasons.

You'll need your workout sheet to record the weights, reps, sets, etc., that the client is performing. Record all of your client's workouts. If you have several clients, this makes it easier for you to remember who did what. Clipboards can be purchased at office supply stores that are hollow, allowing you to house several workout sheets, pens, etc. The information you track for clients can be valuable as a motivational tool down the road. Workout sheets are pretty easy to make on the computer. You can also download templates from the Internet.

If you are working in a health club, you're going to have to share the road with not only the other trainers but also the other club members. Most people in health clubs are pretty courteous to each other and don't mind sharing equipment. If you encounter a member resting on a piece of equipment that you want to use, simply ask the member if you can "work in." Most times people will comply. If you will be using equipment like dumbbells, medicine balls, etc., return them to their proper place before moving to another exercise. Leaving unattended fitness equipment out in the open is a safety hazard.

To Touch or Not To Touch?

Personal training is *personal* and there may be times when it is necessary to touch the client in order to spot them or put them in the right alignment to perform the exercise correctly. It is important to remember that some people may not feel comfortable being touched by another person, especially someone that they hardly know. Touching someone who is not prepared to be touched or feels the touching was inappropriate could lead to disciplinary action or worse yet — legal action! I personally have encountered fitness trainers who do not touch *any* of their clients because of the stigma attached to it. Having said this, it is a good idea to explain the nature of spotting/occasional touching during the initial interview to familiarize the person with the process. During your sessions, when you feel that touching is necessary, ask first if it is ok. In reality, there is no perfect way to address this situation that is right for everybody. I believe that by conducting oneself in a professional manner and by forming true friendships with clients are two of the best ways to reduce any problems from arising from this practice.

When you're working with a client make sure that he/she can exit the machine or exercise safely. When I used to work in health clubs, I would occasionally see trainers who seemed determined to quickly get to the next exercise before the client. They did this probably because they wanted to provide the best service to their clients and get the next station ready for them when they arrived. This is very good but keep in mind that clients may not be as familiar with fitness equipment as trainers. Some fitness machines are pretty complicated and people may have difficulty getting out of a piece of equipment. This can be particularly true for people with special needs, like seniors, those with fibromyalgia or those who are overweight.

It's important to remember that when working with a client he/she should have your undivided attention. This can sometimes be a challenge, especially if you work in a busy health club setting where other members may approach you to ask your advice about something. Undoubtedly, this is a situation that many trainers have wrestled with at some point. Some clubs may try to deal with the situation by having the staff wear different colored shirts to alert members to who is the *fitness floor staff* and who is working in the capacity as a personal trainer. Regardless, if you're working with someone and are approached by another member, be courteous and tell them that you can help them when you are finished with your client. If the need is immediate, refer them to the fitness staff who is on duty.

When you have completed your session with the client, set a date for your next meeting if you have not already done so. Record the date in your day planner. If you are seeing clients back-to-back, give yourself a few minutes between appointments. That will give you time to prepare for the next person. Because it's likely you will be touching various pieces of equipment during the day, it's a good idea to wash your hands between clients. Fitness equipment may harbor germs.[20] Hands should be washed for at least 30 seconds in warm/hot water and soap. If washing isn't possible, carry an alcohol-based sanitary product with you. This may seem overkill to some; however, you would not want to transmit infections to your clients would you? Also, as all personal trainers know, if they don't work they don't get paid. What happens if you get sick? Play it safe and wash/disinfect your hands between clients.

Chapter 3

HOW WILL YOU BE PAID?

Let's now talk about how you will be compensated for personal training. As a rule personal trainers tend to either work in a health-club-like setting or are self-employed. Let's discuss each separately to give you a better idea what to expect.

Working in a Health Club

If you are working at a health club there is a good chance that the client will pay the club and you will receive a percentage of that amount. Only rarely do clients pay health-club-based trainers directly. Clubs usually pay every two weeks. You will probably have to keep track of the number of sessions you have with each client and submit that to the club in order to be paid. You may want to use a day planner to help you keep track of the personal training sessions you perform. I like a day planner that shows me one week at a time. That way I can see what I have to do during a week. This helps reduce the chances of anything sneaking up on me that might be listed on another page. Payment by health clubs for personal training can vary from place to place but usually a couple of scenarios occur:

1. You get a straight percentage (e.g., 50%) of what you generate
2. Your percentage depends on the number of sessions you conduct during the week

As a general rule, health clubs tend to pay 40%-65% of the amount collected to the personal trainer. For example, if the client paid the club $300 for 10 sessions with you and the club paid you 50%, you would receive $150 for that client. Usually, health clubs do not automatically pay you the full amount all at once, but rather for the number of sessions that you perform with that client during the pay period. For example, if you met with the client three times during the previous pay period, you would be paid only for those three sessions. It is in the club's best interest to do this because it helps to protect the club's members. For example, if the club paid the trainer all of the money up front and the trainer quit, the club – and the client – would be at a loss.

Another popular option in some health clubs is to base the trainer's compensation on the number of sessions he/she performs during the pay period. Under this scenario, trainers who worked the most sessions are rewarded for their efforts by receiving a greater percentage than those who worked fewer sessions. From the club's standpoint it's in their interest to do this because it stimulates competition among trainers and gets them to work harder to bring in more money for the club. On the surface it's a good model but the drawbacks are more work for fitness trainers which could lead to greater levels of burnout from spending so much time working. Some clubs may even do away with the traditional "hourly" personal training session and cut it down to 30-minute sessions. The advantage of this is that a trainer could see more people during the day, which, in theory, might mean more money for the trainer.

Another way fitness trainers can be compensated is based on their experience. In other words, the more education, certifications you have, the higher your pay rate. Under this system a trainer who had a BS degree, two certifications, and who also attended regular continuing education seminars, might receive more money than someone who only had a college degree and one certification. In the club's eyes, the more education one has, the more valuable that person is to the organization. In addition, fitness trainers who are also managers may receive higher rates for personal training than non-managers. Managers may also receive yearly *bonuses* for productive work they do in their department as well.

Your compensation rate for personal training will probably be re-evaluated at least twice a year. During this meeting, bring all of your certifications, awards and continuing education certificates. Bring also any degrees you have. If you have testimonials from clients, bring them as well. The bottom line is that the more valuable you are to the club, the higher your pay rate will be.

Another factor that influences how much you make as a personal trainer is whether you receive an hourly rate of pay in addition to personal training compensation. Sometimes the personal training rate you receive may be less because you are a salary-based employee. If you are receiving a salary the odds are good you are also getting health insurance benefits. In this instance the club might cut back on what you get for personal training to compensate. In other words, they see you more as an employee and less as a personal trainer. On the other hand, sometimes your personal training rate may be higher because your hourly rate is low or you're not working many hours at the club. Perhaps you are only officially working in the club 10 hours a week. Because this probably doesn't amount to much money, the club might sweeten the deal by giving you a higher percentage of any personal training revenue you generate.

However you are paid, sit down with the club's manager, personal training director or direct supervisor and have them specifically iron out exactly how you will be compensated.

Self-Employed Personal Trainers

Personal trainers who are self-employed typically charge more per session than health clubs. This is because as a self-employed personal trainer you must pay for everything. This includes the equipment you use, the clothes you wear, liability insurance, health insurance, gasoline and even wear and tear on your car. Many times you may also travel to people's homes for personal training.

The rates of self-employed trainers vary from place to place. It really is true what they say: Location. Location. Location. Trainers in affluent areas may charge hundreds of dollars for a single session while those in less well-to-do areas may make a lot less! Typically, though, sessions will range somewhere between $50-$150 per session. According to the US Bureau of Labor and Statistics, the average annual income for personal trainers and group fitness instructors was about $25,000 in 2004. They go on to say that about 10% of those trainers make about $60,000 per year and the income for self-employed personal trainers can be much higher still. These numbers depend not only on location but also your ability to sell the benefits of your knowledge and expertise to people as well as any other complimentary services/products you offer.

The reimbursement methods for personal trainers who are self-employed differ significantly from those employed in health clubs, most notably because clients will pay them directly. As a self-employed trainer you have several options: cash, check or credit card. Also unlike trainers who work in a health club setting, self-employed trainers usually receive all of the money up front. They then recharge the client when the agreed upon sessions have been completed. Being paid with cash has the advantage that it's immediately usable. You don't have to go to the bank first because the money is in your hand. One disadvantage is keeping track of who paid you what. If several people paid you different amounts in cash you're going to have to remember who paid you which amount. Another disadvantage of insisting on cash is that people generally may not have large sums of cash on hand on a regular basis. Also, unlike other payment methods, if you lose the money, it's gone. Lastly and most importantly, remember that even though it's cash, you must still pay state and federate government taxes on that money.

Another option is to be paid by check. This is a popular method because it's easy to do for most people. The disadvantage is that you usually have to keep informing the client that their session payments are depleted and it's time to renew.

The last payment option is to obtain the privilege of accepting credit cards. You do this by getting a *merchant account*. The major advantage here is that their credit card can be charged again when their session payments are completed. If you are going to accept credit cards there are some things you have to be aware of. The first thing is you need to have a good credit rating. If you do not know your credit rating, you are entitled to a free report each year from the major credit agencies. If you've failed to pay loans or bills on time or declared bankruptcy, these will be red flags that might hinder your ability to obtain a merchant account.

How to Get Your Credit Rating For Free

By law the major credit reporting agencies have to provide you with one free report each year. All you have to do is ask for it. You can obtain your reports by going to this website: annualcreditreport.com. This is a 100% free service that was set up by the three major credit reporting agencies.

Keep in mind that when you accept credit cards, there will probably be a monthly fee associated with this. The monthly fee usually fluctuates with the number of credit card transactions you process each month. The transactions you process will also be subjected to a small fee. In addition, some companies may have an initial set up fee when you apply.

Tips for Getting a Good Credit Rating

---

1. Pay your bills on time
2. Don't skip payments on credit cards
3. Pay *at least* the monthly minimum on credit card purchases
4. Don't max out your credit cards
5. Avoid signing up for too many credit cards

Several organizations can help provide you with a merchant account. Shop around for the one that best suits your needs. Check with your local bank and also go online. Searching online for "merchant account" should return several companies that provide this service.

Keeping Track Of Your Finances

Whether you're self employed or you work at a health club you should make an effort to know where your money is going. This can help you see if you are making money or losing money. For self-employed fitness trainers, this is a no-brainier because you probably have a lot of tax deductions. Even if you work in a health club it makes sense. One of the easiest ways to do this is to get a computer-based money program. All major financial software programs now let you connect directly to your bank via the Internet. This means that the bank will automatically download all bills and deposits you make. All you have to do is spend a couple of minutes to sort them into their proper categories. Having the proper categories is the secret to effective money management.

There is also a good chance that some of your expenses will be paid for in cash. If you are paying for business-related items in cash you can keep track of those as well. You can use your financial software or you can create a spreadsheet. For example, your spreadsheet might look like this:

Business-Related Cash Expenses

March 2009		
	Business Expense	**Amount**
10/1/09	Ink for printer	$ 19.99
10/5/09	Printer paper	$ 10.00
10/15/09	Financial software	$ 39.99
10/21/09	Book: Nutritional Supplements: What Works and Why	$ 24.95
Total		**$94.93**

Keep all your business-related cash receipts, tolls, etc. and add them to the sheet as needed. At the end of the month print the sheet up and put it in the file for that month. Your accountant can use this information when he/she does your taxes.

Self employed trainers who travel to people's homes might have a similar program for their work-related mileage. For example, the spreadsheet might look something like this:

Business Miles Driven

October 2009	Location Traveled To	Tolls	Round Trip Mileage
10/1/09	Bill Leinhauser	$ 3.00	30
10/16/09	Tim DiFelice	-	25
10/27/09	Paul Coppola	0.75	25
Month Total		**$ 3.75**	**80**

Again, you can make a sheet like this for each month in the year. At the end of the year, tally up all the tolls and miles driven for business. Your accountant can use this information when tax time arrives.

If you go to the bank to make deposits and have more than one source of income, use a different deposit slip for each check. This way you'll know how much each client paid you as well as how much you made from other sources of revenue. You won't know this answer if all the deposits are lumped together.

Chapter 4

HOW WE MAKE ENERGY

The classic definition of energy is the *ability to do work*. Work is anything that you do. For example, reading these words, walking and lifting weights are all work and all require energy. As many know, we make energy from the food we eat. For the most part, our energy comes from carbohydrates and fats, with proteins normally used to a much lesser extent. However, less well-known is that before we can utilize the energy within the macronutrients (calories), it must first be transformed into a type of energy that we know how to use. For humans, this ultimate energy molecule is called *adenosine triphosphate* (ATP). This is actually very similar to how your car works. Your car does not run on oil. Rather the oil has to be refined into gasoline before your car can use it. The same is true for us. We take the raw materials in food and refine them into a *gasoline* that we understand how to use. The process of making energy is technically called bioenergetics. This chapter will review the major ways that we can make energy and relate those process to exercise.

What Does ATP Look Like?

The ATP molecule essentially looks like this:

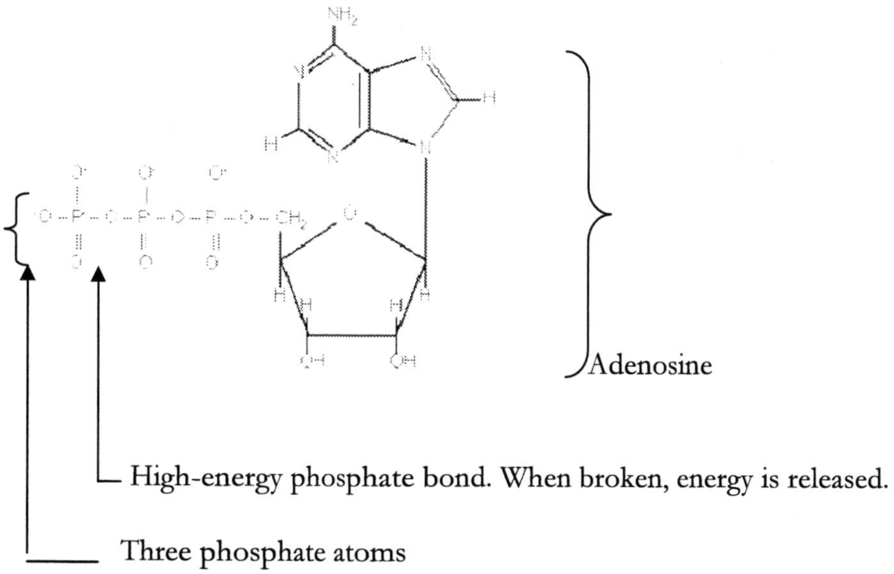

Adenosine

High-energy phosphate bond. When broken, energy is released.

Three phosphate atoms

As can be seen from the picture, ATP is made of a molecule of adenosine (a type to sugar) and three phosphate atoms. The short lines between the phosphate atoms represent chemical bonds. There is energy within these bonds. The chemical bond attached to the last phosphate is called a "high energy bond." When this bond is broken, much energy is released. This is the energy that powers our activities. The breakdown of ATP is accomplished via an enzyme called an ATPase. When ATP loses its high energy phosphate it becomes adenosine diphosphate (ADP). From here, ADP can further break down to adenosine monophosphate (AMP). Neither ADP or AMP is specifically relevant to the scope of personal training so they will not be discussed.

Making Energy: The Big Picture

The process of making energy (ATP) is complicated but basically we have two ways of accomplishing this task. One of those ways uses oxygen to make energy and is called the *aerobic energy system*. The other way does not need oxygen to work. It is called the *anaerobic energy system*. You can think of these energy systems like gears in your car. We have a *gear* inside of us that works at lower intensities of activity and tends to burn a lot of fat. This is the aerobic energy system. The other gear we have works at higher intensities of activity and tends to burn a lot of sugar (carbs). This is the anaerobic energy system. Unlike the gears in your car, however, our gears —aerobic and anaerobic — are always working inside of us. In other words, we are never only burning fat and we are never only burning sugar. Rather, we are, for the most part, always burning some mixture of fats and sugars to power our energy needs. At lower intensities of activity, we tend to burn greater percentages of fat, while at higher intensities of activity, we tend to burn greater percentages of sugar.

Another important thing to remember is that it is not only the *intensity* of activity that dictates what we burn for fuel but also the *length of time* that we can do the activity. In other words, if you can perform an activity for a long time, you are burning a large percentage of energy from fat to do that task. If you can only perform the activity for a short period of time, carbohydrates (e.g., glucose) are supplying the bulk of your energy needs. Reading these words is pretty easy and right now about 30%-40% of the energy that lets you do this is coming from carbohydrates. The other 60%-70% is coming from fat.[77] This is why you may have read that low intensity exercise burns fat while high intensity exercise burns sugar. While this statement is true, some misinterpret it to mean that the best way to burn fat is to do low intensity exercise. We will address this issue separately. Let's now discuss the aerobic and anaerobic energy systems in greater detail.

The Macronutrients

Food	Calories / Gram[*]
Protein	4
Carbohydrate	4
Fat	9

* There are 28 grams in once ounce.

The Aerobic Energy System

The term aerobic literally means "living in oxygen." One of the most popular names for the aerobic system is the *Krebs cycle*, named in honor of its discoverer, Hans Krebs. Alternative names include the *citric acid cycle* and the *tricarboxylic acid cycle* (TCA cycle). Still another more technical name is *oxidative phosphorylation*. The Krebs cycle is a complex series of chemical reactions that essentially results in energy (ATP) being produced from the breakdown of fat. This is why people who are trying to lose weight are often counseled to perform aerobic activity —because the Krebs cycle uses oxygen to burn fat. The Krebs cycle occurs within the *mitochondria*. Just as our bodies have different organs, the cells of our bodies also have organs that do specialized tasks. The mitochondria are one of the many *organs* of your cells and one of their main jobs is to burn fat. Biology teachers often call mitochondria the "powerhouses of the cell" because a lot of energy is produced from the breakdown of fat. In reality the mitochondria are like batteries. Just as a battery can produce electrical energy, mitochondria produce biological energy and do so in a very similar way to the batteries in your car, mp3 player, etc. Thus, mitochondria are essentially aerobic, rechargeable, fat burning batteries!

Human Cell

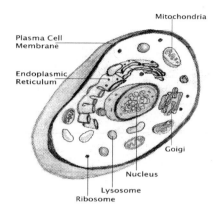

Until now we have discussed just the Krebs cycle; however there is another series of chemical reactions that occurs inside the mitochondria. This other chemical reaction series is called the *electron transport chain* and it is from this that the battery analogy stems from. The bottom line of the Krebs cycle and the electron transport chain is that each glucose molecule burned can result in the generation of 38 ATPs. Carbon dioxide and water are produced in the process.

While a single glucose molecule can produce 38 ATPs, it turns out that the aerobic. breakdown (oxidation) of fat can yield even more energy! Fat is technically called a fatty acid or *triglyceride*. A triglyceride is basically three long chains of carbon atoms anchored to a glycerol molecule. When fat is broken down, it first enters a chemical reaction called *beta oxidation* which chops the fat up into smaller parts. These parts are transported to the mitochondria with help of a taxicab molecule called carnitine. The smaller bits of fat then enter the Krebs cycle and electron transport chain where they produce ATP. It turns out that hundreds of ATP molecules can be produced from a single triglyceride molecule. Like the end products of glycolysis, carbon dioxide (which we exhale) and water are also produced.

With respect to exercise, aerobic exercise training causes the mitochondria of exercising muscles to enlarge and become more numerous. Bigger, more numerous mitochondria can burn more fat. So we would expect to see bigger and more numerous mitochondria in the muscles of a triathlete, cyclist or bodybuilder (bodybuilding does have an aerobic component). Often, those not accustomed to exercise exhaust themselves rather quickly. One reason for this is that their mitochondria are smaller and less numerous. Thus, they are not good at fat burning. In this instance, their bodies rely more heavily on burning carbs (glycogen and glucose) anaerobically. This results in the build up of lactic acid (lactate) that plays a role the characteristic burning sensation inside muscles that forces the person to cease exercise. Aerobically trained muscles, on the other hand, use more fat and less glycogen during exercise. Since the depletion of carbs (glycogen and glucose) can greatly hinder exercise performance, this means that exercise-trained muscles can work longer because of their lower reliance on carbs and greater reliance on fat. This helps us exercise longer because we have a limited ability to store carbs in the body and if those carbs were exhausted, exercise would stop, like your car stops when it runs out of gas. We store enough carbs to run for about 20 miles. On the other hand, the average person has enough energy in the form of fat to run for almost 1000 miles! While all energy systems are always working inside of us, in general, the aerobic energy system begins to contribute significantly to our energy needs during activity lasting longer than 3 minutes.[78]

The Fat-Burn Program

Because low intensity activities that we can do for long periods of time, burn greater percentages of fat, many treadmills and other pieces of cardio equipment have a "fat burn" program. Essentially this program holds people at a relatively low percentage of their maximum heart rate (~60%). While we do indeed burn more fat at lower intensities of activity, it may not always be the best for weight loss. For example, as one walks slower, a greater percentage of fat is used. Sitting burns more fat than standing. Technically, sleeping is the greatest fat burning activity with about 70% of the energy coming from fat breakdown. So, why doesn't anyone lose weight sleeping? What people who use the fat burn program may not realize is that they don't use many calories in this mode of exercise. Calories are the key to weight loss (and weight gain). Sleeping doesn't foster weight loss because it doesn't burn many calories. The advantage of the fat burn program however, is that it reduces the risk of injury during exercise. So, for beginners or those with special needs (e.g., overweight), lower intensity is generally best and safest.

The Anaerobic Energy System

The anaerobic energy system basically has two parts: the *ATP/CP system* and *glycolysis*. The ATP/CP system (adenosine triphosphate /creatine phosphate system) is sometimes called the *phosphagen system* because phosphate is common to both compounds. ATP is needed for all activity (exercise and otherwise) to occur. However, we do not store large amounts of ATP in the body. In fact, it's estimated that the body only stores 80-100 grams (3 - 4 ounces) of ATP at any given moment.[8] This is only enough energy for a few seconds of activity. This is why ATP must be constantly made throughout our entire lives.

When exercise demand is very great, creatine phosphate is activated. *Creatine Phosphate* (CP or phosphocreatine) is used to replenish ATP at rates faster than all other aerobic and anaerobic mechanisms. In this way, CP acts like a turbocharger for ATP production. During the regeneration process, CP donates its phosphate atom to ADP to reenergize ATP. ATP then, once again, breaks down, releasing the energy we need. Keep in mind that CP itself cannot provide energy. Only by helping reenergize ATP is CP able to contribute to our energy needs. Generally, our cells can store four to six times more CP than ATP.[8] This extra energy boost from CP can provide about an extra 10-20 seconds of activity during high intensity exercise.[8]

$$CP + ADP \rightarrow ATP$$

It is important to remember that the creatine energy source is not being used significantly during activities that the body feels are low intensity. Thus, in general, CP is not used during activities like walking, hiking, swimming, Yoga or circuit weight-training. Rather, CP is used during heavy weight lifting, sprinting and Karate to name a few. Creatine supplementation will further be discussed in the *Questions and Answers Chapter*. For more information on creatine and more than 100 other supplements, read my book, *Nutritional Supplements: What Works and Why*, available at www.Joe-Cannon.com.

The other part of the anaerobic system is *glycolysis*. Glycolysis refers to a series of chemical reactions in our cells in which ATP (energy) is made via the anaerobic breakdown of carbohydrates. Glycolysis is also sometimes called the *lactic acid system*. This refers to *lactic acid* (lactate) a metabolic byproduct formed during glycolysis. The fuel of choice used in glycolysis is the sugar, glucose. Glucose is a simple sugar (monosaccharide) the body prefers to use and is the reason it is often called "blood sugar." In fact, some organs of the body (e.g., the brain) must have glucose to function.

Lactic Acid and Muscle Fatigue

Lactic acid (also called lactate) production, correlates with reduced ability to perform strenuous exercise. For example, increased lactic acid levels reduce the pH of cells (i.e., makes them more acidic) which aggravates nerve endings, causing feelings of pain and burning inside the muscles. More specifically it is the rise in hydrogen atoms within the cells that causes the burning and pain rather than lactic acid itself. Measuring lactic acid levels however provides an indicator of hydrogen atom concentration. The rise in lactic acid levels (and hydrogen atoms) reduces our ability to make ATP via glycolysis and inhibits the strength of the myosin/actin cross bridge binding. This in turn inhibits the force production of muscles. Lactic acid production however does not result in muscle pain the next day (DOMS), given that most of the lactic acid has been removed from the cells about an hour or so after exercise. Likewise, lactic acid is not a waste product. After exercise, some of the lactic acid is transformed into glucose and stored for future use.

During glycolysis, glucose is sent through a series of chemical reactions, which results in the creation of ATP (energy). Specifically, 2 ATPs can be made per glucose molecule (3 ATPs if we use glycogen). In addition a byproduct called *pyruvate* is also made. Pyruvate, in turn, has the opportunity to be converted to a similar molecule called *lactic acid* (lactate) which is linked to muscle fatigue and the burning sensation felt during intense exercise. Pyruvate may also take another path as well. In the case where exercise is easy enough that sufficient oxygen is present, pyruvate does not become lactic acid but rather is transported to the mitochondria and converted to another compound (acetyl coenzyme A) which helps to make even more ATPs via the Krebs cycle. This alternative route is sometimes called *aerobic glycolysis* because oxygen is used to help further metabolize pyruvate to make more ATP molecules. Those struggling with this concept and wondering which aspect of glycolysis—aerobic or anaerobic—occurs during different types of activities should remember that at higher intensity activity (when ATP must be made fast), anaerobic glycolysis predominates. During lower intensities of activity (when ATP doesn't need to be made as fast), aerobic glycolysis and the Krebs cycle are more likely to occur. Generally speaking, glycolysis tends to contribute significantly to our energy needs during exercise lasting 2-3 minutes.[78] After that, the aerobic energy system starts to prevail.

It is important for fitness professionals to understand that when carbohydrates are eaten, they are chemically rearranged into glucose. Glucose, in turn, is stored in the body in the form of another molecule called *glycogen*. When needed, glycogen is brown down to glucose which then enters cells and can be made into energy. Thus, glucose and glycogen are basically the same thing. The formation of glycogen from glucose is called glucogenesis. Conversely, the breakdown of glycogen to form glucose is called glucogenolysis. One major difference between glycolysis and the Krebs cycle is that glycolysis occurs inside the watery-like cytoplasm of the cells. The Krebs cycle, on the other hand, occurs in the mitochondria, which floats within the cytoplasm.

The Lactate Threshold

The lactate threshold is the point during exercise when lactate levels begin to rise dramatically in the blood. In other words, it is the point or threshold when one begins to rely heavily upon the anaerobic energy systems to sustain exercise. Another term which means same thing is lactate inflection point (LIP). For those who are accustomed to exercise, this threshold is usually reached at about 70%-80% Karvonen HR max (~70% - 80% VO2max) and at ~50-60% Karvonen HR max for untrained person's.[78] It turns out that if exercise continues to increase beyond this point, another inflection point occurs where lactate levels rise even further. This second threshold is called the onset of blood lactate accumulation ("OBLA"). According to some, this second threshold corresponds to the body's greater reliance on type II muscle fibers which are recruited in greater numbers to help sustain the exercise intensity.[78]

For athletes, training at intensities close to or at lactate threshold or OBLA may help the body better deal with lactate clearance and increase the intensities at which these thresholds occur. In theory, this may help athletes exercise at higher intensities without dealing with significant lactate accumulations. Those seeking general cardiovascular benefits do not have to worry about these thresholds. Rather, moderate activity of 20-60 minutes most days of the week will suit their needs fine.

Exercise Intensity and Duration: Which is Aerobic and Anaerobic?

Exercise Intensity & Duration	Energy System Used
High Intensity, Short Lasting	Primarily anaerobic
Low Intensity, Long Lasting	Primarily aerobic

Which Sports Use Which Energy System?

In general, it can be said that any activity that one can perform for a long time is using the aerobic energy system to a greater degree than the anaerobic system. Conversely, any activity that one can only perform for a short period of time is primarily utilizing the anaerobic system. The following are some examples of activities and the energy systems they are primarily using:[24]

ATP/CP System mostly	ATP/CP & Glycolysis	Glycolysis mostly	Glycolysis & Krebs cycle	Krebs Cycle mostly
100 m sprint	200 m sprint	400 m sprint	800 m sprint	Triathlon
1RM lift	Baseball homerun	Tennis	Boxing	Marathon
Diving	Basketball	100 m swim	Rugby	Jogging
Jumping	Ice hockey sprint	Soccer	1 mile run	Cross country skiing

It should be stressed that, in reality, the fitness level of the person really determines which energy system is being used. In other words, it is possible for an activity that is traditionally considered to be aerobic to be perceived by an untrained person to be anaerobic. Some people may be so unfit (e.g., old age, sarcopenia, disease) that walking a few yards taxes the aerobic system more than it can handle, resulting in the person to rely heavily upon anaerobic energy mechanisms. This, in turn, would cause that person to run out of steam sooner than expected.

Protein Use and Exercise

As a rule, protein contributes about 2%-10% of our energy needs, although others estimate its rate of breakdown can be as much as 20% in some extreme instances.[86] Protein use is likely to be elevated with long duration exercise (e.g., a marathon) especially in person's with poor diets. Two key nutrients that help us preserve protein are adequate calories and carbohydrates. In the absence of enough calories (e.g., dieting) protein may be broken down to help create energy to make up for what is no longer being consumed. Specifically, protein can be transformed into glucose via gluconeogenesis. The glucose produced can be used for energy. Athletes sometimes supplement with branch chain amino acids (BCAA) because they can be burned for energy inside muscle cells.[38] The BCAAs are leucine, isoleucine and valine. Other studies hint that these amino acids may help reduce fatigue during exercise.[38] Less well-known to people is the role that carbohydrates play in helping preserve muscle. Carbohydrates can help prevent protein from being broken down just as BCAA supplements might. For those on a budget, carbohydrates may be a cheaper alternative.

What Happens After Exercise?

After the cessation of exercise, the energy that has been expended must be replaced. For example, lactic acid that accumulates during exercise can be transformed into glucose and stored as glycogen via a series of chemical reactions called the Cori Cycle. It turns out that energy expended via the anaerobic energy systems are reenergized via the aerobic energy system. More specifically, after exercise, people will continue to breathe deeper than normal for a period of time. The extra oxygen that is consumed helps the aerobic system replenish the energy stores used during anaerobic exercise. This is sometimes called the *oxygen debt*. A more descriptive term for this is *excessive postexercise oxygen consumption* (EPOC). Another way of thinking of this is that it refers to the elevation of metabolic rate that occurs after exercise has stopped. Both aerobic and anaerobic exercise elevates EPOC —but which does so the most? This will be addressed in the *Question and Answer* chapter.

Practical Applications

Fitness professionals should have a working knowledge of energy systems because this can help them train their clients according to the client's needs and goals. Remember, the body responds specifically to the exercise demands placed upon it. For example, those who want to improve sprinting performance should focus on developing their anaerobic energy systems. Many sports involve various combinations of all the energy systems, so the job of the trainer is to figure out the best mix for the client. Whatever the person's goal, however, it is wise to begin the program at a low intensity and progress to the desired level of fitness over time.

Chapter 5

ANATOMY AND PHYSIOLOGY

The Planes of the Body

Movement can occur in different orientations or planes. The planes in which movement can occur are the sagittal plane, the frontal plane and transverse plane.

Sagittal plane. Imagine a vertical line going through the body and breaking it up into both left and right sides. This is the sagittal plane.

Frontal plane. Imagine a line cutting the body into two parts – front and back. This is the frontal plane.

Transverse plane. In this plane, a line divides the person into an upper and lower part. An analogy to this would be a magician who "saws" a lady in half.

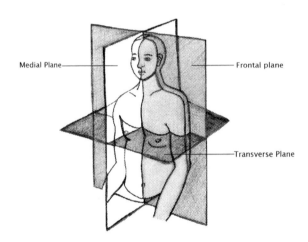

It's important to remember that while three planes of movement are usually discussed, human movement patterns in everyday life sometimes involve two or more planes at once. This gives rise to the term *triplanar*. Triplanar movements are more real-life. This, in turn, gives rise to the popular term *functional* which refers to movement patterns that better mimic what a person does in the real world. For example, getting up from the floor is more functional than using the leg press machine. In essence, functional exercises train movement patterns, not necessarily muscles.

Common Anatomy Terms

Medial. Medial refers to being close to the midline of the body. If you were performing internal shoulder rotation you would be rotating your arm medial or toward the body.

Lateral. Lateral refers to being farther away from the body. Lateral also refers to movement away from the midline of the body. If you were doing external shoulder rotation, you would be moving your arm lateral from the body.

Proximal. Proximal refers to being close to a reference point or the midline of the body. For example, the humerus is more proximal to the shoulder than the radius bone.

Distal. Distal refers to something being situated far from its point of origin or reference point. For example, the foot is more distal from the head than is the nose.

Pronation. Turing your hand such that your that palm is facing downward. For example, if you perform a reverse biceps curl, you do so with your hands in the pronated position. With respect to the feet, pronation occurs when the foot is oriented such that the inner portion of the foot is rotated inward. The prone position also occurs when you lay face down.

Supination. Refers to rotating your hands so that your palms are facing up. The biceps is responsible for supination and this is why some supinate their hands as they lift dumbbells; the thought being that if you combine both actions of the biceps (elbow flexion and supination) that you would stimulate the biceps to grow more.

Superior. This term usually refers to being above a reference point. For example, the head is more superior to the heart than the feet. The *superior vena cava* returns blood to the heart from the upper portion of the body.

Inferior. Inferior refers to being below a reference point. For example, the femur bone is inferior to the ribs. The *inferior vena cava* returns blood to the heart from the lower portions of the body.

Anterior. This term refers to being in front or before the body, organ or reference point. For example, the anterior deltoid is the front portion of the deltoid muscle group. Anterior is the opposite of posterior.

Posterior. Refers to being behind a reference point or located toward the rear. It is the opposite of anterior. For example, the back of the shoulder is often referred to as the posterior deltoid.

Plantarflexion. This term usually refers to the foot and is used when the foot is bent such that the toes are pointing straight ahead. Imagine a dancer on her tippy toes.

Dorsiflexion. This term usually refers to the foot and is used when the foot is bent such that the toes are brought close to the body. Walking on your heels requires you to dorsiflex your feet.

Tissues of the Body

A *tissue* is a group of cells that performs a specific function. Generally speaking, four groups of tissues are usually discussed: epithelial tissue, nerve tissue, connective tissue and muscle tissue.

Epithelial tissue is essentially single cell layers of tissue that serve many different functions. For example, epithelial cells line the insides of your blood vessels (i.e., endothelial cells) where they ensure proper, turbulent-free movement of blood, while epithelial cells on the surface of your skin act as a barrier between you and the outside environment.

Nerve tissue conducts electrical impulses between the brain and the rest of the body.

Connective tissue serves a number of purposes such as forming tendons and ligaments as well as providing an overall structural framework to the body. Bone, blood and fat are all connective tissues. Another connective tissue called cartilage can also act as a shock absorber between bones.

Muscle tissue allows us to not only interact with the outside environment but survive as well. If it were not for the heart, arguably the most important muscle, none of us would be here! Muscle tissue can be further subdivided into three types: smooth muscle, cardiac muscle and skeletal muscle. *Smooth muscle* lines blood vessels and allows them to expand and contract when needed. *Cardiac muscle* is heart muscle. One of the main differences of cardiac muscle and others is that its contraction is involuntary. In other words, we do not have to think to make the heart contract. This is good news because if we had to think in order to get the heart to contract, none of use would last very long. *Skeletal muscle* is the type that is usually of most interest to fitness professionals. It is called skeletal muscle because, for the most part, it is attached to the skeleton (e.g., biceps, quadriceps, etc.).

Organs are specialized tissues that do specific tasks. For example, the heart, kidneys, brain, skin and lungs are all organs. A *gland* is a specialized type of organ that produces a substance (e.g., a hormone) that is released into the blood or body cavity. Generally, two types of glands are usually recognized: *exocrine* glands and *endocrine* glands. Exocrine glands secrete substances into a duct or passageway that is close to where it is located. Examples of an exocrine gland include mammary glands, sweat glands and salivary glands. Endocrine glands, on the other hand, generally secrete substances (e.g., hormones) into the blood where they can then travel far from their place of origin. For example, the beta cells of the pancreas make the hormone, insulin, which travels through the blood and help cells process sugar (glucose) and amino acids.

Examples of Endocrine Glands and the Hormones they Produce

Gland	Selected Hormone Made	Function
Adrenal glands	Adrenaline (epinephrine)	Fight or flight response
Pineal gland	Melatonin	Sleep
Pituitary gland	Growth hormone	Growth and various other functions
Thyroid gland	Thyroid hormone	Regulates metabolism
Pancreas	Insulin and glucagon	Decreases and increases blood sugar respectively
Kidneys	Erythropoietin (EPO)	Makes red blood cells
Liver	Insulin-like growth factors (IGFs)	Various functions
Skin	Vitamin D	Improves calcium absorption
Testes	Testosterone	Muscle growth and other functions

Two other examples of endocrine glands that may not be apparent yet, of interest to fitness professionals are fat cells and the stomach. Fat cells (adipose cells) secrete a hormone called *leptin* that plays a role in eating. In essence, when leptin levels are high (e.g., after eating), it sends a signal that we are full. When leptin levels are low, the signal is that we are hungry.[49] Another hormone is ghrelin, made in the stomach. High levels of ghrelin stimulate appetite while low levels reduce appetite.[50] It is important to remember that while leptin and ghrelin play roles in eating and gaining weight, they are not the only players in the game. People eat for a variety of reasons. Fitness professionals should ask for peer-reviewed evidence for any nutritional supplement touted to promote weight loss by blocking or inhibiting either of these hormones.

Connective Tissue and Cartilage

Connective tissue is a general term for a diverse type of tissues that serve many different functions. Blood, bone, tendons and cartilage are all examples of connective tissues which help the body function properly. Cartilage is one of the most prevalent connective tissues in the body and helps form joints, ribs, tendons, ligaments and ears. Because of its dense nature, cartilage is able to sustain great forces without being damaged. This makes cartilage perfect for the ends of the long bones of the body where it helps reduce friction and serves as a shock absorber. During the disorder, *osteoarthritis*, however, this cartilage is damaged which results in pain as bones grind together. Cartilage is avascular which means that it has no direct blood supply. This is why tendons and ligaments take so long to heal after they are injured. One component of cartilage that helps give the tissue its strength is chondroitin sulfate. Chondroitin sulfate is also marketed as a dietary supplement to help osteoarthritis.[38] The evidence for this supplement helping arthritis though is uncertain.[38]

Essentially two types of cartilage are generally discussed: fibrous cartilage and hyaline cartilage. *Fibrous cartilage* is sturdy and found in tendons and ligaments as well as in the disks of the spinal cord. Conversely, *hyaline cartilage* is found in areas like the trachea (wind pipe) and at the ends of the long bones of the body (e.g., femur). The hyaline cartilage found at the ends of bones is often called *articular cartilage* or joint cartilage (articular means joint). This is the cartilage that is worn away in osteoarthritis.

Tendons

A tendon is a tough band of connective tissue (mostly collagen) that usually connects muscles to bones. When muscles are worked, the force of that activity is transmitted from the muscles to the tendons which in turn pull on the bone. This is why it's possible for resistance training to also strengthen bones and help offset osteoporosis. In other words, as you strengthen muscles you also strengthen bones.

At the point where the tendon and muscle come together (called the myotendinous junction) is a specialized sensor called the *Golgi tendon organ* (GTO). The GTO monitors force production by the muscle. If the GTO senses that the muscle is producing so much force that it or the tendon might be damaged, the GTO activates. When this happens, the GTO *relaxes* the muscle! In extreme instances, the GTO may also even cause the contraction of the antagonistic muscle to further help reduce injury! You can think of the GTO as a safety mechanism that protects the body from harm. Many people outside of fitness are unaware of the GTO. This, coupled with the desire to lift heavy weights, has the potential for serious injury. For example, consider a novice who is performing very heavy bench presses without a spotter. This person lifts so much weight that the GTO activates. The GTO "thinks" that an injury to the muscle or tendon is about to occur. It doesn't "know" that the person has 300 pounds suspended above his/her body! In this situation the muscle relaxes and the barbell falls onto the person, causing serious, possibly life-threatening injury. This is why it's always recommended that people use the buddy system when lifting weights. Fortunately, by employing *progressive overload resistance training*, muscles, tendons and ligaments all grow stronger over time which, in turn, resets the point at which the GTO activates. This is why it's possible for some people to lift tremendous amounts of weight.

Muscle Spindles

Related to the GTO is another type of receptor called the *muscle spindle*. Muscle spindles reside within the muscle and relay information about the length of the muscle as well as the speed of change in muscle length. When the muscle spindles *sense* that a muscle is stretching too fast, they send a signal to the CNS which in turn relays a signal back to the muscle to contract! In this way, muscle spindles protect muscles from being stretched too far or too fast. With respect to stretching, this is why it's recommended to not stretch too fast or to the point of pain. Stretching to the point of pain (or stretching too fast) activates the muscle spindles which in turn contract the muscle, defeating the purpose of stretching! This phenomenon is sometimes called the "stretch reflex." Muscle spindles are essentially modified muscle fibers and are sometimes called *intrafusal fibers* to differentiate them from the *extrafusal muscle fibers*, (i.e., slow and fast twitch fibers) which generate force and power. Both muscle spindles and GTOs are referred to as *proprioceptors*, specialized sensory receptors that monitor and relay information about motion or body position.

Tendon placement can also play a role in how strong a person is or can be. Thus, where a tendon attaches to the bone can dictate how much force the muscle associated with that tendon can produce. This in turn might play a role in how big muscles might get from strength training. Tendon placement is genetically predetermined and cannot be altered significantly by training.

Ligaments

Like tendons, ligaments are also made of tough connective tissue that is mostly made of collagen. Unlike tendons, which connect muscles to bones, ligaments connect the bones together. When one bone is connected to another, a *joint* is formed.

Joints

A joint is formed when two bones come together. Another term for joint is *articulation*. The disorder known as arthritis is one that affects the joints. *Osteoarthritis* (abbreviated as OA or DJD), the most common form, occurs when the cartilage cushioning between joints wears away. The type called *rheumatoid arthritis* (abbreviated RA) occurs because of an autoimmune disorder whereby the immune system attacks the joints of the body causing inflammation and pain. There are different joints of the body and each type serves different purposes and has a different range of motion (ROM). The shape of the bones, the toughness/tightness of the ligaments and even the arrangement of muscles around a joint can impact the joint's ROM. Some people claim to be 'double jointed." Often, this situation is caused by ligaments that are not as tight as "normal" joints. A dislocation (luxation) can occur when one of the bones forming a joint is out of place. A subluxation is a partial or incomplete dislocation. Common signs of a dislocation can include swelling and/or pain in the joint that follows an activity and/or loss of motion at the joint.[133] A synovial joint is one of the most common and is called such because of the synovial membrane that covers the joint. The synovial membrane makes a fluid (synovial fluid) that helps reduce friction. The shoulder, wrist, knee and elbow all contain synovial joints.

The Human Skeleton

The skeleton can be divided into two parts. They are the axial skeleton and the appendicular skeleton. The *axial skeleton* is composed of the skull, vertebral column, sternum and ribs. The *appendicular skeleton* is composed of the long bones of the upper and lower body (humerus, radius, ulna, femur, fibula and tibia) as well as the scapula, clavicle and pelvis.

Human Skeleton: Front View

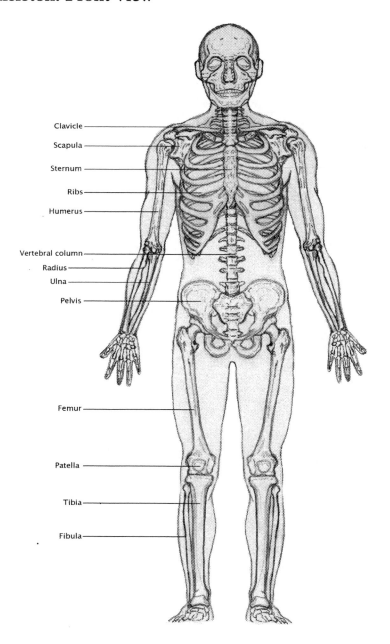

Clavicle

Scapula

Sternum

Ribs

Humerus

Vertebral column

Radius

Ulna

Pelvis

Femur

Patella

Tibia

Fibula

Human Skeleton: Rear View

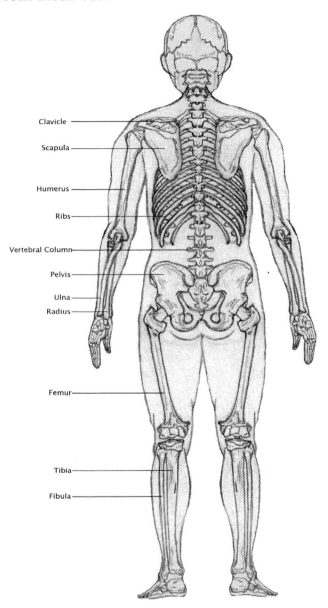

Clavicle

Scapula

Humerus

Ribs

Vertebral Column

Pelvis

Ulna

Radius

Femur

Tibia

Fibula

The Spinal Column

From top to bottom, the major sections of the spinal (vertebral) column are called cervical, thoracic, lumbar, sacral and coccygeal. There are 7 *cervical* vertebrae (numbered C1 to C7); 12 *thoracic* vertebrae (numbered T1 to T12); 5 *lumbar* vertebrae (numbered L1 to L5); 5 *sacral* vertebrae (numbered S1 to S5) and 3 to 5 fused bones in the *coccygeal* area. The coccygeal area (also called coccyx) is sometimes called the "tailbone" because of thoughts by some that it's a leftover from an earlier evolutionary stage in our development. Experts estimate that more than 90% of low back problems occur in the lumbar spine, specifically in the area called L5-S1. That is, the 5th lumbar vertebrae and the 1st sacral vertebrae.

Bone

There are 206 bones in the adult human body and they make up about 20% of the body weight of an adult. Besides providing a scaffolding for the body, bones also act as a reservoir for minerals (e.g., calcium) if needed. The bone marrow is also where red blood cells (RBCs) are formed.[24] Small bones in our ears are also primarily responsible for our ability to hear. Bone is actually a living tissue that is constantly undergoing growth, repair and degradation processes. Bone can be divided into two forms: cortical bone and trabecular bone. Cortical bone is dense and compact and forms the hard, outer shell of bone. Trabecular bone (also called cancellous bone or spongy bone) is softer and is found inside bone but also adds to bone strength.

There are four types of bones in the body: long bones, short bones, flat bones and irregularly- shaped bones. The bone shaft of long bones is called the *diaphysis* and the ends of these bones are called the *epiphysis*. It is at the ends of long bones (epiphysis) that long bones grow longer. These regions are called the *epiphysial plates* (growth plates). Growth plate damage is often cited as a reason to dissuade kids from lifting weights. While possible, especially with maximal and/or overhead lifts, research also finds that *supervised* resistance training can also help reduce injuries in adolescents.[77]

The process of bone formation is called *osteogenesis* (*osteo* means bone). Bone growth and repair is complex; however, three types of cells are usually described. They are osteoblasts, osteocytes and osteoclasts. *Osteoblasts* are essentially baby bone cells. Osteoblast cells begin bone formation by making several proteins and related compounds including collagen, calcium carbonate and calcium phosphate. These become the *matrix* of bone. Eventually the matrix hardens, giving bone its strength. Because the matrix of bone is related to its strength, health professionals often discuss a concept called *bone mineral density* (BMD). The greater the BMD, the stronger the bone is.

Osteoblast cells eventually become mature bone cells called *osteocytes*. Cells called *osteoclasts* degrade bone. As osteoclasts degrade bone, its minerals (e.g., calcium) are released for the body to use if adequate nutrients are not consumed in the diet. Ultimately, this process can lead to bone being degraded faster than it can be made, resulting in a loss of BMD. Eventually, this process can make bones porous and weak, leading to *osteoporosis* (brittle bone disorder). This is why an unhealthy diet is partially linked to osteoporosis. Fortunately, because muscles are attached to the bones it is possible for strength training to help counteract osteoporosis. It's important for fitness professionals to remember that osteoporosis is not simply a condition that affects people who are "old." Long-term bed rest, various diseases or just not moving enough can all lead to reduced bone density. Men also get osteoporosis. Some evidence hints that the greatest rate of bone loss occurs within the first seven weeks of no physical activity.[41] Since there is no gravity in outer space, astronauts, may be at greater risk of osteoporosis.[41]

Chapter 6

MUSCLE PHYSIOLOGY

The human body has over 600 skeletal muscles. Interestingly, muscles are only able to *pull*. No muscle can push anything. It is only because of the intricate interactions between different muscles and their associated bones that we are able to perform pushing actions. This chapter will deal with various issues related to muscle physiology that fitness professionals should be familiar with. This chapter is by no means comprehensive. Indeed, people have devoted their entire lives discovering how muscles work and many fine books have been written solely on this topic. The goal of this chapter is to cut to the chase and provide the fitness professional with relevant information without going into the nitty gritty details that usually never pop up in conversation with the general public.

Surface Muscles: Frontal View

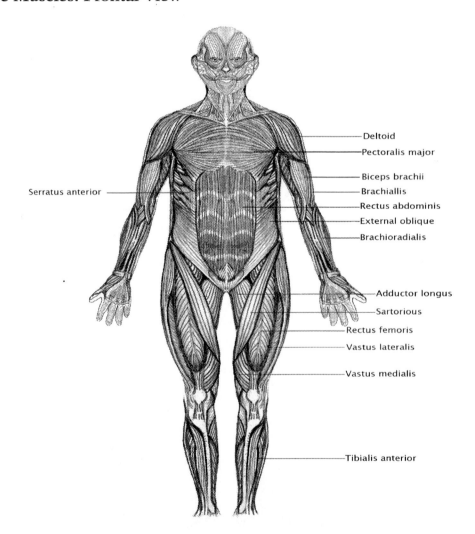

Deltoid
Pectoralis major
Biceps brachii
Brachiallis
Rectus abdominis
External oblique
Brachioradialis
Serratus anterior
Adductor longus
Sartorious
Rectus femoris
Vastus lateralis
Vastus medialis
Tibialis anterior

Surface Muscles: Rear View

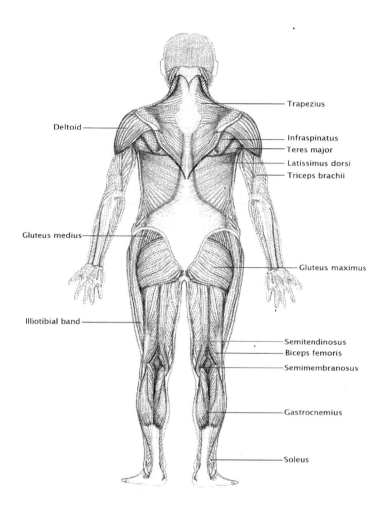

Deltoid

Trapezius

Infraspinatus

Teres major

Latissimus dorsi

Triceps brachii

Gluteus medius

Gluteus maximus

Illiotibial band

Semitendinosus

Biceps femoris

Semimembranosus

Gastrocnemius

Soleus

Basic Muscle Physiology

Since fitness professionals deal continuously with muscles it is important that they have a grasp of how muscles work. Let's now discuss the basic structure of a muscle fiber. Muscles are of course made of muscle fibers, also called muscle cells. As mentioned previously, muscles are attached to bones by way of tendons. If you could pull one of your muscle cells out of your body you would see that it was covered by a connective tissue called the *epimysium*. In fact, tendons are basically extensions of the epimysium that reach out and grab onto bones. Looking deeper into a muscle we would see that the fibers are bundled into groups called *fascicles*. These, in turn, are covered by connective tissue called the *perimysium*. Each muscle fiber that makes up a fascicle is, in turn, further covered by connective tissue called *endomysium*.[24] It is important to remember that each connective tissue layer – epimysium, perimysium and endomysium is basically an extension of the tendon.[78] Thus, when a muscle develops force, that force is transmitted back to the tendon, which, then pulls on the bone. This is how strength training the muscles is able to strengthen bones. The membrane that surrounds each muscle fiber is called the *sarcolemma*.[24]

As mentioned previously, a fascicle is a group of muscle fibers (muscle cells). If we could pull out one of the fibers that make up a fascicle we would see that the fiber is made up of even smaller units called *myofibrils*.[78] Myofibrils, are composed of a variety of myofilament proteins needed to foster muscle contraction. Two of these proteins are myosin and actin. *Myosin* is a thick protein. *Actin* is a thinner protein. These myosin and actin proteins are stacked or layered on top of one another inside myofibrils and give the fibers a striped appearance and make up the force generating functional unit of muscle contraction —the *sarcomere*. When a muscle contracts, it is the sarcomeres which make up that muscle fiber that actually contract. During the contraction process, actin and myosin protein filaments slide over each other. This leads us to the next topic – the *sliding filament theory* of muscle contraction.

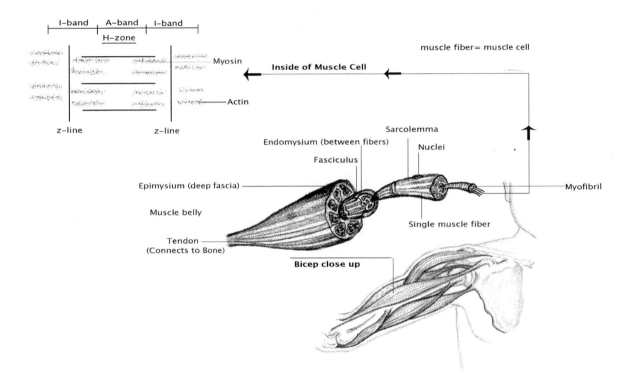

The Sliding Filament Theory

The process that best describes how our muscles function is referred to as the *Sliding Filament Theory* of muscle contraction first postulated in the 1950s.[29,41] According to this theory, the actin and myosin proteins (myofilaments) are contained within *sarcomeres*, which are the basic unit of muscle contraction. Muscle cells are made up of many sarcomeres which are layered or stacked on top of each other.

When stimulated to contract, the actin and myosin filaments literally slide over each other as a muscle is worked. More specifically, the thin, actin proteins are pulled by the thick myosin proteins in what has been described by some as a ratcheting motion. This is made possible because the myosin proteins have, jutting out from them, globular heads that are able to make contact with the actin proteins. You can think of these myosin globular heads as looking like the heads of a golf club or hockey stick. They are able to form a bridge that travels across from the myosin protein to the actin proteins. This bridge from myosin to actin is technically called a *cross bridge*. When stimulated by nerve impulses, the globular head of the myosin cross bridge attaches to its corresponding attachment site on the actin protein and pulls it. It then releases and reattaches itself to another attachment site along the actin protein and pulls again. As this ratcheting process (called *cross bridge cycling*) continues, the muscle shortens and contracts, generating the force it needs to perform work such as standing up, walking, dancing, or curling a barbell, for example.

The energy that powers the cross bridge on myosin to pull the actin filaments during muscle contraction is supplied by ATP. Myosin proteins contain an enzyme (called a myosin ATPase) that breaks down ATP, releasing the energy needed for cross bridge cycling to occur.[22] It's interesting to note that APT does not directly cause myosin to pull actin. Rather, ATP is needed for the myosin cross bridge to detach from its attachment site on the actin filament. After it detaches from one site, it is able to reattach to another site and pull actin once again.

Can We Run Out of ATP?

While exhaustive exercise may diminish ATP levels for a short time, they are never depleted entirely. The body is very good at continually producing ATP through both its aerobic and anaerobic energy systems. In fact, if we were not able to make ATP, we would die! *Rigor mortis*, one of the earliest signs of death, occurs when the muscles become rigid and not easily moved. This phenomenon is due to the inability of the body to produce ATP any longer. In the absence of ATP, the myosin cross bridges are basically "frozen" to the actin filaments, causing the rigid appearance indicative of rigor mortis.

Recall that we have different types of muscle fibers – type I (slow twitch) and type II (fast twitch). It turns out that the fast twitch fibers have a myosin ATPase enzyme that breaks down ATP faster than slow twitch fibers.[41] The faster ATP can be broken down means the faster that cross bridge cycling can occur – which means the faster the muscle can contract. This is why fast twitch fibers are called fast twitch.

Obviously, the sliding filament theory is a lot more complicated than what was just described. For example, we still call it a theory because nobody has ever seen living tissue contract at the molecular level. For more in-depth reviews on these and other topics, see the references.

The Brain/Muscle Connection

The fact that we must think before skeletal muscle does anything means that there is a connection between the muscles and our brain. Let's now talk about that connection and how it works.

The process that describes how a nerve impulse induces a muscle contraction is referred to as *Excitation-Contraction coupling* because it couples or connects the excitatory (stimulating) signals of the nervous system with the contracting muscles. When we make a conscious decision to move a muscle, the impulse starts in the brain, in an area called *primary motor area*. It is here that an excitatory brain chemical called a neurotransmitter, (e.g., acetylcholine) is released from a brain cell (neuron) and travels over to another brain cell, which in turn regenerates the nerve impulse (called an *action potential*). This process continues from cell to cell until the signal reaches the muscle. It is important to note that the stimulus needed to obtain a nerve impulse must be of sufficient strength before an impulse is created. This makes sense, otherwise any stimulus we encounter during the day could lead to muscle contractions or other involuntary reactions. Only after an impulse crosses this threshold is an action potential generated.

The regeneration of the nerve signals from one brain cell to another is accomplished because the neurotransmitter is able to alter the concentration of sodium and potassium (electrolytes) within the cells. More specifically, when the neurotransmitter reaches another cell it causes the potassium to temporarily leave the cell, while at the same time, allowing sodium to temporarily rush inside the cell. The effect of this is that the electrical nature of the cell momentarily transforms from electrically positive to electrically negative. It is this temporary electrical depolarization of cells that allows nervous impulses to travel throughout the body.

When the nerve impulse reaches the muscle, it first makes contact with the gap or space between the nerve cell and muscle cell (called the *neuromuscular junction*) and from here, travels across that space to the muscle cell. Upon reaching the muscle cell the impulse first makes contact with muscle cell membrane (sarcolemma) where it again causes alterations in the concentration of sodium and potassium, (i.e., sodium enters the cell while potassium exits) which, in turn, further spreads the impulse over the muscle cell, like water spreading out over a table. The action potential (nerve impulse) then travels down into the muscle cell by way of channels called the transverse tubules (*T-tubules*). This stimulates a portion of the cell called the *sarcoplasmic reticulum* (SR) which contains calcium. When stimulated by the nerve impulse, the sarcoplasmic reticulum releases calcium into the cell. Before we go any further let's introduce two additional muscle proteins called *troponin* and *tropomyosin*, which sit on the actin protein molecule and are important for regulating how actin and myosin interact. Essentially, troponin sits on top of tropomyosin. This blocks the myosin attachment site when the muscle is relaxed. When calcium is released from the sarcoplasmic reticulum, it diffuses through the cell and makes contact with troponin. This causes the troponin to shift its position and in doing so moves tropomyosin out of the way, revealing the actin attachment sites so the myosin cross bridges can bind, facilitating muscle contraction.

Obviously, it would not be good for muscles to be constantly contracted, so there must be a way for muscles to relax. Remember that the sarcoplasmic reticulum releases calcium into the cell. The SR has cellular pumps which remove calcium from the cell and return it to its storage site. As calcium levels fall within the cell, the troponin-tropomyosin complex returns to its resting state, once again blocking the attachment sites on actin causing muscles to relax.

What are Motor Units?

Muscle fibers (muscle cells) are stimulated by nerves. The nerves that stimulate movement are called motor nerves or motor neurons. They are also sometimes called *alpha motor neurons*. A *motor unit* refers to a motor neuron (brain cell or nerve) and all the muscle cells that it directly stimulates.[30] The motor nerves (*motor* refers to movement) send electrochemical signals from the brain, down the spinal column which eventually end up at muscle cells. In this way, the brain is able to tell a muscle to contract. When a motor unit is stimulated, all of its associated muscle fibers contract. Different muscles can have different numbers of motor units. In general, the more precise the movement, the fewer muscle fibers are stimulated by a single motor unit. For example, the eye muscles may have very few muscle fibers associated with a motor unit while a biceps muscle may have thousands of fibers per unit. Most muscles have hundreds to thousands of motor units associated with them.[41] The more motor units that are activated, the more muscle fibers are stimulated and hence the greater the muscle contraction. Lifting a heavy weight will recruit more motor units (and a more forceful muscle contraction) than lifting a lighter weight.

Studies show that motor units come in different sizes and that the smaller motor units are recruited first followed by larger motor units. This rule is often referred to as the *Size Principle*.[52]

Smaller motor units are recruited first because the impulse needed to activate them is less than that needed by larger motor units.[52] Another way of saying this is that smaller motor units stimulate slow twitch, type I fibers while larger motor units stimulate fast twitch, type II fibers. It is because of the size principle that type I fibers are always recruited first, followed by type IIa and then type IIb. This actually makes sense. For example, if you were carrying this book to your car, you would want to use only your type I fibers. If you instead used your type IIb fibers, they might fatigue before you reached your car and you'd drop the book!

Delayed Onset Muscle Soreness

The feeling of pain or discomfort in muscles in the hours and days following a strenuous or unaccustomed activity is called *delayed onset muscle soreness* or "DOMS" for short. Anything that's intense enough or that you are not used to doing will cause DOMS if you do it long enough. This can be anything from shoveling snow from your driveway to going out and running around the block one time. The pain usually occurs 24 to 72 hours following exercise. The soreness usually subsides within 7 to 10 days of the soreness-initiating event. Muscles during this time are said to be stiff and there is often a decreased range of motion. During this time, people report a lowered ability to produce force in the affected muscles. Thus, people may not be able to lift as much when they experience DOMS. Research has shown that this is the result of both a decreased ability of the muscle to produce force and an unwillingness on the part of the person to use the DOMS-affected muscles.[115] Interestingly, DOMS is not felt when the muscle is at rest; rather, we only feel the pain when the muscles in question are worked or when the muscles are touched.[116] This fact can sometimes help fitness trainers to differentiate between DOMS and some other more serious types of pain (e.g., tendonitis). In other words, failure to experience pain when not moving may be a tip off that the person is experiencing DOMS.

DOMS does not result in any long-term damage to muscles. However, there is evidence of short-term damage. Muscle biopsies during DOMS reveal damage to key areas of muscle structure.[117] For example studies show physical damage to sarcomeres as well as to their associated connective tissues and elevations in various enzymes associated with tissue injury.

There are several theories to explain why DOMS occurs. All theories have merit; but, no theory fully explains the process. The most common theories are the torn tissue theory, connective tissue theory and inflammation theory.

Theories of DOMS

Theory	Main Details
Torn Tissue Theory	Damage to muscles is cause of DOMS
Connective Tissue Theory	Damage to connective tissue is cause of DOMS
Inflammation Theory	White blood cells release chemicals that sensitize pain receptors

The theories aside, what everyone agrees upon is that eccentric activities (e.g., walking downhill or lowering a dumbbell.) or "negatives" as they are often called, result in far more DOMS than concentric movements.[119]

Some may take various drugs like aspirin or other non-steroidal anti-inflammatory drugs (NSAIDs) to alleviate DOMS. While this practice can help reduce pain it may not be the best practice for elite athletes. There is evidence that NSAIDs reduce protein synthesis following eccentric exercise.[120] This, in theory, might prolong DOMS and reduce athletic performance. For most people, however, this effect is probably not significant.

One common misconception about DOMS involves lactic acid. There is no proof that lactic acid causes DOMS. People who say this probably confuse muscle burning during exercise with muscle pain (DOMS) the next day. They are not the same thing.

Another common misconception about DOMS involves stretching. To date there is not much evidence that stretching sore muscles alleviates DOMS. In fact, there is evidence that stretching can cause DOMS, if you are not used to stretching.[118] Stretching between sets however may speed recovery during subsequent sets. Likewise, the impact of various nutritional supplements (e.g., antioxidants) to protect against DOMS or speed relief has, at best, mixed results and is not fully accepted.[38] As for so-called sports creams, these mask pain with either sensations of heat or cold. They do not speed recovery from DOMS. Currently, the only accepted therapy for reducing DOMS is performing a submaximal bout of the exercise before the actual workout.[122] In other words, do one set of an exercise a day or so before doing 3 sets. In practical terms, novices who perform one set and gradually build upon this over time are less likely to experience DOMS or more serious injuries than those who partake in more aggressive exercise routines.

Types of Muscle Fibers

There are basically three types of muscle tissue in the body: smooth muscle (in blood vessels), cardiac muscle (in the heart) and skeletal muscle (biceps, triceps, etc.). This section will deal only with skeletal muscle.

Skeletal muscle is called *skeletal* because, for the most part, it's attached to the skeleton. Skeletal muscle is also called *voluntary* muscle because we voluntarily cause it to move. For example, the biceps muscle can't automatically lift a dumbbell; we must first think, "Lift that dumbbell," before it happens.

What About Heart Muscle?

Skeletal muscle and cardiac (heart) muscle have similarities; however, one important difference is that cardiac muscle is *involuntary*. In other words, we don't have to think to make it contract. Imagine the problems we would have if we always had to concentrate on keeping our heart beating!

Skeletal muscle can be further divided into *type I muscle fibers* and *type II muscle fibers* and various subtypes of each. The type I and type II fibers are also sometimes called slow twitch and fast twitch muscle fibers respectively, where the "twitch" refers to contraction speed (in other words slow twitch fibers twitch or contract slower than fast twitch fibers). The type II fibers can be further subdivided into different subtypes. Usually we discuss *type IIa fibers* and *type IIb fibers*. Let's explain each in more detail now.

Type I muscle fibers are small fibers that produce low amounts of force, but they can produce that force for long periods of time. Thus, type I fibers are hard to fatigue. This is because they are aerobic fibers that contain an abundance of myoglobin (an oxygen-carrying molecule similar to hemoglobin), mitochondria and capillaries which allow them to burn fat and glucose for energy. They are purely aerobic fibers and generally do not have the ability to work anaerobically. With respect to exercise, type I fibers do not show as much hypotrophy as other fiber types and are used during activities that are not overly difficult. They are called type I because they are usually the first muscle fibers that are activated when a muscle contracts. They are also called slow twitch fibers because they contract slower than fast twitch fibers (about 110 milliseconds vs. about 50 milliseconds for type II fibers). Another term for type I fibers sometimes used in academic settings is *slow oxidative* fibers. This term is more descriptive, referring to both the fibers' slow twitch properties as well as their ability to oxidize (i.e., burn) fat/sugar aerobically. Type I fibers used to be called "red fibers". This is because they are rich in mitochondria which contain red-colored pigments called cytochromes.

Type IIa muscle fibers are "middle of the road" fibers. They are not only larger than type I fibers (but smaller than type IIb) but they also generate much more force. They also are able to produce force for longer periods of time. These fibers are used during a variety of activities such as resistance training, hiking, sprinting, etc. Thus, type II muscle fibers are both aerobic and anaerobic. While sometimes called fast twitch, another term used is *fast oxidative glycolytic* (FOG). This term makes reference to their ability to burn fat and sugar aerobically and anaerobically. They also utilize the creatine energy system.

Type IIb fibers are the most powerful fibers in the body. They contract the fastest of all known fiber types. But, the power they produce doesn't last long. Thus, type IIb fibers are also the quickest to fatigue and have low endurance.[52] Two reasons for this is that they have the lowest number of mitochondria and capillaries (both of which are needed to burn fat). Type IIb fibers are strictly anaerobic fibers and basically use glucose (and creatine, depending on the intensity of activity) to generate force. Because they are fast twitch and rely upon glycolysis and other anaerobic means to generate force, they are sometimes called *fast glycolytic fibers* (FG). These fibers have the thickest diameter. They are also used during activities that are perceived as very demanding such as powerlifting, bodybuilding (depending on the load lifted), sprinting, etc. It's important to note that fitness level dictates what is easy and difficult. For some people, getting out of a chair is very difficult! Interestingly, new research suggests that, with exercise training, type IIb fibers begin to take on characteristics of type IIa fibers.[62,77] This may be the body's way of adapting to exercise. In other words, type IIa fibers are more useful than type IIb in that they are almost as powerful and can do a lot of things type IIb can't.

Quick Reference

Muscle Fiber Type	Brief Description
Smooth muscle	Lines blood vessels.
Cardiac muscle	Heart muscle. Also called involuntary muscle because it can contract on its own.
Skeletal muscle	Mostly attached to skeleton. Also called voluntary muscle.
Type I muscle fibers	Aerobic fibers. Endurance fibers. Burn fat and glucose.
Type IIa muscle fibers	Both aerobic & anaerobic. Strength & endurance fibers.
Type IIb muscle fibers	Totally anaerobic. Power fibers. Fatigue very fast.

People may have had problems naming muscle fibers in the past because different books may call them different terms. The following table sorts through the confusion.

Muscle Fibers Types. Old Names and New Names

Commonly used name	Commonly used name	Older name	Technical name
Type I fibers	Slow twitch	Red fibers	Slow Oxidative fibers (SO fibers)
Type IIa fibers	Fast twitch	Pink fibers	Fast oxidative glycolytic fibers (FOG fibers)
Type IIb fibers	Fast twitch	White fibers	Fast Glycolytic fibers (FG fibers)

How Many Muscle Fiber Types Do We Have?

It appears that humans possess many different subtypes of muscle fibers besides type I and type II that are normally discussed. For this reason, some may read about other fiber types including type IIAB, type IIx and type IIc. These other types can be thought of as hybrids of the major types. However in fitness, we usually only discuss type I, IIa and IIb fibers.

How Many Type I and Type II Fibers Do We Have?

It is sometimes stated that adults have roughly 50% slow twitch and 50% fast twitch fibers. The problem with this statement, though, is that it is practically impossible to prove. Intuitively, it makes sense that people are blessed with both endurance and strength/power fibers. But, the only way to really confirm this is to cut the muscle open and biopsy it. Since there are over 600 muscles in the body, this is not ethically possible to do. What we can say is that different muscles tend to have different percentages of type I and type II fibers. For example, the abdominals tend to have high concentrations of slow twitch, type I fibers while the leg muscles tend to have higher concentrations of fast twitch, type II fibers. Also, there is research that some endurance athletes have greater concentrations of type I fibers while some strength and power athletes may have more type II fibers.[53] Thus, genetics plays a role in fiber distribution. Other research of biopsied muscle also has noted that young men tend to have more type IIa fibers in their vastus lateralis while women tend to have more type I fibers.[54] The bottom line is that people have both type I and type II fibers. How much of each can vary and is open to speculation.

Some have tried to devise ways of estimating muscle fiber type dominance by way of exercise.[55,56] One method is based on first determining 1RM and then performing as many reps as possible using 80% of 1RM.[57] If the person can perform more than 12 reps then that muscle group is said to be composed of at least 50% type I fibers. If they can do less than 7 reps, then the muscle group is at least 50% type IIb fibers. If they perform somewhere between 7-12 reps, then the muscle group is supposed to have equal percentages of type I and type II fibers. Recipes like this and others are sometimes cited on websites, but they have not been well-studied clinically.

Do Men Have More Muscle Fibers Than Women?

Generally speaking men tend to be stronger than women because they have a greater overall amount of muscle than women. However, a type I or type II muscle fiber from a woman is the same as that of a man and responds the same to exercise training.[62,76] It also appears that men and women have relatively the same percent of type I and type II fibers per muscle group.[76] Women do tend to be weaker in upper body strength relative to men but that has more to do with men having greater upper body muscle density than their fibers being stronger.[76] Because of the fiber type resemblance between genders, it is generally not necessary to train women differently than men.

Can Women Get Big Muscles?

Thoughts of getting large muscles, like that of a man, have unfortunately discouraged more than one woman from lifting weights. However, this will not happen for the vast majority of women because most do not have enough anabolic hormones (e.g., testosterone) which facilitate muscle growth. While there are very muscular woman in the world (e.g., female bodybuilders) they usually have to train for many years, lifting very heavy weights to get this big. These women also eat a lot more calories and protein than most. Others may also have genetic advantages like naturally higher levels of testosterone or higher percentages of type II muscle fibers. Still others may use anabolic steroids. Sometimes overweight women will describe how they "get big" from strength training. This may be due to their slightly enlarged muscles expanding the overlapping adipose tissue (fat), giving the impression that their muscles have grown greatly in size. Reducing calorie intake and adding some aerobic exercise should help reduce adipose girth. While it is possible that the muscles of some women may exhibit hypertrophy, this is outside the norm. For the most part this should not happen.

Can Exercise Alter Muscle Fiber Type?

Is it possible that exercise can change type I fibers into type II fibers (or vice versa)? While there is some research to suggest the answer is yes, the degree of change and significance of these changes is controversial.[41] One study of untrained person's who participated in high intensity, intermittent cycle sprints noted an increase in type IIa fibers with a decrease in type I fibers.[58] Since type IIa fibers have some attributes in common with type I fibers (endurance ability) it's likely that this apparent switch resulted from modifications in chemical composition between fibers rather than one fiber transforming into another. Currently there is no real proof that exercise training can change a type I fiber into a type II fiber.[62] People who are usually interested in this question are athletes. However, athletic performance is not just about fiber type. Practice and determination are also involved. As evidence of this, remember that one of the greatest athletes of all time — Michael Jordan — was once cut from his high school basketball team!

Can We Make More Muscle Cells?

The technical term for making new cells is *hyperplasia.* While the main process whereby muscles grow bigger and stronger is by *hypertrophy*, there is evidence that under some conditions we may be able to make more muscle cells. Most of the support for hyperplasia stems from animals subjected to long periods of stress (example, stretching for 30 days straight!)[59] With respect to humans, some controversial research of highly trained bodybuilders finds larger muscles (i.e., triceps) than in non-bodybuilders while the size of individual muscle fibers between the two groups was not different.[60] This hints that hyperplasia may occur under some stressful exercise conditions. Not all studies though, are in agreement with this finding.[61] Other possible lines of evidence for hyperplasia include *satellite cells* (undifferentiated proto-muscle cells) and *muscle fiber splitting*, where one muscle cell splits into two. What can be said for now is that if hyperplasia of muscle cells occurs, the process of how to make it happen is open to speculation. Also, because it has not been directly observed in humans, its impact on muscle size and strength may not be significant and limited to activity that is intense in nature. So, while hyperplasia can't be ruled out, the vast majority of evidence finds that hypertrophy (increase in size) of muscle cells is the major way muscles grow bigger and stronger.[29]

Atrophy

Muscle atrophy, refers to loss of muscle size and strength. In most people, atrophy begins to occur after about three weeks of not working out; however, for highly trained athletes, it may occur sooner.[41] During this process, muscle proteins begin to break down at a faster rate than protein synthesis. Eventually this results in a loss of strength. This lack of strength coupled with an increase in connective tissue (that contributes to muscle stiffness) intermixed between muscle fibers makes it difficult for people to perform activities of daily living (ADLs), resulting in depression, loss of productivity and, if taken to its ultimate conclusion, confinement to a nursing home. Exercise – especially weight bearing and/or resistance training – is one of the best ways to combat muscle atrophy. When prescribing activities to reduce atrophy fitness professionals should consider the limitations of the client and, if possible, design activities that overload weakened muscles just a little more than they are used. Activities that duplicate ADLs can also be great help in improving this condition.

Besides reduced exercise habits, atrophy can also result from poor nutrition, inadequate calories (and protein) eating disorders, lack of anabolic globally-acting hormones (e.g., testosterone or GH), reduced nervous stimulation to an area, too much bed rest and even spaceflight to name a few. In addition, various diseases (cancer, COPD, etc.) also result in muscle atrophy. Because so many conditions can lead to atrophy, the fitness professional should consider this when evaluating his/her clients.

Conditions Where Atrophy May Be Observed[*]

Inactivity	Sedentary jobs	Anorexia Nervosa	Poor nutrition
Cancer	HIV/AIDS	Bulimia	Inadequate protein
COPD	Prolonged bed rest	Burns	Depression
Immobilization	Parkinson's disease	Stroke	Aging process
Arthritis	Prednisone therapy	Injury	Diabetes

*Not a complete list

Sarcopenia

In general, people gain strength up to the age of 30, after which it slowly begins to decline.[66] First coined in 1989, *sarcopenia* is a type of atrophy that refers to the age-related loss of muscle size and strength.[63] After age 30 people tend to lose 0.5 % of their muscle mass per year until the age of 50.[66] After 50 the loss of muscle accelerates.[65] While all muscle fibers are affected by sarcopenia, one of the most salient features of this condition is that it almost exclusively targets type II muscle fibers.[67,69] This probably is at least partially related to the reduced use of these fibers as people age (i.e., use it or lose it). This almost preferential loss of type II fibers has profound implications for loss of mobility and independence as we get older and fitness professionals should have an understanding of this process so that they can not only recognize sarcopenia but help people deal with it better. It is important to make the distinction between sarcopenia and other similar conditions fitness trainers may have heard about like *muscle wasting* and *cachexia*. Muscle wasting refers to muscle loss resulting from lack of use or disease. It can occur at any age and is usually what is referred to as "atrophy." In adults, a BMI of less than 18.5 sometimes indicates muscle wasting. Cachexia on the other hand is more frequently associated with disease, such as cancer. Sarcopenia is different from these in that it is specifically related to the aging process.

Atrophy Conditions: How They Differ

Muscle wasting	Atrophy stemming from disuse
Cachexia	Disease-induced muscle and weight loss
Sarcopenia	Age-related muscle loss

Both men and women get sarcopenia; however, some research hints that men (possibly because of their greater muscle mass) may experience sarcopenia to a greater degree than women.[63] For example, some research has noted that 58% of men over the age of 75 had sarcopenia compared to 45% of women of the same age. However, because women tend to live longer, they may be at greater risk of experiencing the ravages of sarcopenia for longer periods. Currently, why sarcopenia occurs is unknown and there are likely many factors that lead to this condition. One factor we have no control over is genetics. Sarcopenia may be programmed into us and is a part of the aging process. Reductions in anabolic hormones may also be involved. Also, muscle fiber stimulation from the nervous system appears to decrease as we get older because of a gradual loss of motor units. Muscle cells that are no longer stimulated will die off. As we age we may also be less efficient at making muscle proteins.[70] Some research finds a 30% reduction in muscle protein synthesis as we age.[65] Myostatin is a protein that reduces muscle growth. Some research finds that myostatin levels rise as we age.[71] As an aside, some supplements are touted to naturally block the effects of myostatin, promising muscle growth without any effort. Fitness professionals should remember that many of these supplements lack proper research to substantiate their claims.[72] For a better understanding of "myostatin blockers" and over 100 other supplements, read my book, *Nutritional Supplements: What Works and Why* available at www.Joe-Cannon.com. Regardless of myostatin's effects, evidence does suggest that resistance training can stimulate protein synthesis in older men and women.[73]

Unlike genetics, how we live our lives also plays a critical role in the development of sarcopenia. For example, lack of appropriate physical exercise probably accelerates sarcopenia. Generally, as people age, they are less likely to engage in resistance training which helps preserve type II fibers. Also, as people grow older, they may avoid tasks that they deem too difficult to do (like weight lifting or carrying groceries). Many older individuals continue to walk as they get older; but walking mostly enlist endurance-oriented type I fibers. The lack of appropriate stimulation (i.e., strength training, particularly eccentric actions) of type II fibers as we age is probably one of the main reasons for their almost selective decline with sarcopenia.

Poor nutrition can also impact sarcopenia. People tend to eat fewer calories and protein as they grow older. In the absence of adequate calories and protein, the body, in an attempt to stay alive, may cannibalize itself to obtain the energy it needs. Gluconeogenesis refers to the creation of glucose from non-carbohydrate energy sources. Protein is a non-carbohydrate energy source. In essence, the body may begin to degrade its own protein, turn it into sugar and burn it for energy. In the absence of proper amounts of exercise, the body may choose to degrade the muscle fibers that are no longer being used – type II fibers. This may be one of the reasons type II fibers are decimated in sarcopenia. As type II fibers dwindle, it becomes even more difficult to perform ADLs. When a person does move, they are slower, which in turn may increase their risk of injury. For example, those with sarcopenia may take longer to cross the street if a traffic light suddenly changes. They may also be less likely to catch themselves if they fall. Fitness professionals should remember that in some older people, the sensation of thirst also may decrease, leading to reduced fluid consumption. This may lead to fatigue, which, in turn, may result in less activity, further advancing sarcopenia.

The loss of strength accompanying sarcopenia can also compromise other aspects of health. For example, sarcopenia may lead to less aerobic activity like walking which may contribute elevations in cholesterol, LDL and triglycerides with corresponding decreases in HDL. Obviously this would exacerbate/promote heart disease.

Because muscle is involved with metabolic rate (the speed we burn calories), sarcopenia may lead to a lower BMR. Some have estimated that from age 30-80 there is approximately a 15% decrease in BMR.[65] This can lead to weight gain, making people even slower and less likely to exercise.

The loss of muscle may also contribute to type II diabetes. Muscle burns more calories at rest than fat. The loss of muscle accompanying sarcopenia means less muscle available to use the calories consumed during a meal. In theory, this means higher insulin levels are needed to store the extra calories as fat. Chronically higher insulin levels might reduce the number of insulin receptors, leading to insulin resistance, metabolic syndrome and ultimately type II diabetes.[67,68] Diabetes further escalates the risk of a number of complications related to heart disease.

Sarcopenia is a term not often mentioned in fitness circles; That being said, it is safe to say that every person reading these words will be impacted by this condition eventually. Considering that America is fast becoming a nation of older people, the ravages of sarcopenia have profound implications for not only the healthcare system but, in this author's opinion, national security as well. By recognizing sarcopenia, fitness professionals, more than any other healthcare specialist, have a unique opportunity to be at the forefront of the public's education of this often overlooked phenomenon.

Sarcopenia May Contribute To

Increased falls	Reduced ability to perform ADLs	Poor quality of life
Reduced strength	Lack of independence	Depression
Slower speed	Confinement to a nursing home	Reduced immune system
Lower aerobic capacity	Reduced metabolic rate	Early death

Types of Muscle Actions

Essentially there are three different types of muscle actions (muscle contractions) that are usually discussed. They are isometric muscle actions, isokinetic muscle actions and isotonic (dynamic) muscle actions. Of these, human muscles usually perform either isometric actions or the more frequently occurring, isotonic muscle actions. Let's now discuss each in greater detail.

Isometric Muscle Actions

The prefix *iso* means "same" and *metric* means distance, so isometric muscle actions occur when no change in muscle length occurs as the muscle is used. In addition, there is also no change in the joint angle during isometric muscle actions. Other names that also refer to isometrics include *static contractions and dynamic muscle tension*. An example of this type of muscle action is if you were to press your hands together in front of your chest as hard as you can or if you were to press against an immovable object like a wall. The core muscles of your trunk also isometrically contract as you perform many of your everyday activities. Isometric muscle actions were popular in the early 20th century but eventually fell out of favor by strength trainers and were replaced by the more popular isotonic muscle actions. Some weightlifter's still incorporate them into their exercise routines. An example of this might be the person who holds the contraction for a second or two at the end of each repetition. Isometrics by themselves will increase muscle strength; but they are less effective than isotonic muscle actions. The reason for this is that the joint angle is fixed in isometric exercises. For example, if you pressed your hands together in front of your chest as hard as you could, your strength would increase; however, if an object was then placed between your hands (adjusting the joint angle), the strength increase would not occur or be less. In other words, by not moving the muscle through its full safe range of motion, strength development over that ROM is less. Another drawback to isometrics is that they tend to raise blood pressure more than other modes of strength training.[47] As such, they are not recommended as the only mode of exercise for people with high blood pressure or heart disease.

Isokinetic Muscle Actions

The prefix *Iso* means "same" and *kinetic* refers to speed or movement. Thus, isokinetic muscle actions are those that occur at the same speed throughout the range of motion. Typically when we exercise, our muscles do not move at a fixed rate of speed, so this type of muscle action does not mimic what we do in real life. Performing isokinetic movements requires the use of equipment such as what may be seen in physical therapy. Indeed, physical therapists may use isokinetic exercises that only allow the muscle to move at a specific speed. The advantage of this type of muscle action is that the muscle can exert maximum force throughout its ROM. Again, while isokinetic exercise can increase strength, its application to real world activities seems limited (remember the principle of specificity). Some healthclubs may have a piece of equipment called an upper body ergometer (UBE) in which the person rotates his/her arms in a circular fashion. One of the settings on the UBE is an isokinetic mode in which you can set the machine to only move at a certain speed. No force you can apply will cause the machine to move faster. The UBE can also be of help during shoulder rehab or can provide an aerobic workout to those who can only use their upper body muscles.

Isotonic (Dynamic) Muscle Actions

This is the type of muscle actions we do most. The term isotonic refers to constant tension being produced inside the muscle and how the muscle length changes as we go through a movement's safe range of motion (ROM). Isotonic muscle actions are composed of two phases – *concentric* and *eccentric*. If we limit the discussion to strength training, concentric muscle actions (sometimes called positives) occur when we are lifting the weight. If we could look at the muscle cell during a concentric muscle action, we would see that the actin and myosin proteins are sliding closer together, which shortens the muscle length. Eccentric muscle actions (sometimes called negatives) usually occur when we are lowering a weight. During eccentric actions, we would observe that the actin and myosin proteins are being pulled apart. Thus, during eccentric muscle actions, the muscle lengthens as force is applied to it.

Eccentric muscle actions can result in greater improvements of strength and higher metabolic rates compared to concentric movements. The downside is that eccentrics also result in a more delayed onset muscle soreness (DOMS).[48] Sometimes people call eccentrics, eccentric muscle *contractions*. However, this is technically a misnomer since a muscle can't contract when it is elongating. This is why you will see the phrase *eccentric muscle actions* used more often.

Types of Muscle Actions: How They Compare

	Isometric	Isokinetic	Isotonic
Joint movement	None	Yes	Yes
Speed of movement	None	Constant	Varies
Force generation	Constant	Variable	Constant
Change in fiber length	No	Yes	Yes

Women's Fitness Centers

Fitness centers that cater to only women have become quite popular, the most notable of which being Curves®. Many women-only fitness centers are unique in that, by the use of specialized hydraulic equipment, they remove the eccentric component of exercise. One of the main reasons for this is that eccentric movements produce more DOMS than concentric movements (though concentrics can cause some DOMS). Many of these centers also make use of circuit training which is efficient, boosts strength and endurance, is not boring and allows one to effectively work her body in 30 minutes or less. This is especially important for beginners and those with tight schedules who cannot devote longer time periods to exercise. With respect to effectiveness, one study of the exercise protocol used by Curves found that a typical 30-minute workout burned between 164 and 238 calories in "unfit" women and 522 calories in "fit" women.[87] By fostering a nurturing, friendly environment and showing people how they can fit exercise into their busy life, women's-only fitness centers have become formidable competition for more traditional gyms and health clubs.

Do Muscles Have a Memory?

The concept of "muscle memory" refers to the phenomenon whereby trained muscles, after a period of non-use (e.g., not working out for a few months) appear to regain their strength at a faster rate than they originally did when training first began. In reality, what is referred to as muscle memory is probably better described as a brain-muscle memory because it is the brain which relays instructions to the muscles to perform a movement. In some circles this type of memory is referred to as *procedural memory* because the brain is remembering how to perform a procedure. For example, we've all heard the phrase "you never forget how to ride a bike." No matter how long it's been since you rode a bicycle, you pick the skill up faster than when you first learned it. With respect to exercise, one study noted that sedentary women who strength trained for 20 weeks, then stopped for 30-32 weeks and then lifted again for six weeks, regained strength faster than it took them to get stronger at the start of the study. [88] In addition, cross sectional area (i.e., the thickness) of type II fibers also increased faster than at the start of the study. The mechanisms behind muscle memory are not well understood, but at least partially, probably involve the interaction of the brain and central nervous system.

Strength Training and Testosterone

Testosterone is primarily produced by the Leydig cells of the testes and to a lesser degree by the adrenal glands. While typically considered a *male* hormone, women also make this testosterone in the ovaries and adrenal glands, albeit to a lesser degree than men. In men, testosterone is usually highest in the morning lowers over the course of the day.[78] Testosterone impacts a number of organ systems, with the muscles being the most notable. Following secretion, testosterone travels through the blood usually attached to a specialized protein (sex hormone binding globulin or SHBG) that acts to inhibit the hormones action.[90] Most of the circulating testosterone is bound to this or other proteins and is not thought to be active. In contrast, about 0.2% - 2% is the active, free testosterone.[90] At its target sites, testosterone binds to testosterone receptors on the cell's surface and, through a complex series of reactions within the cells brain center (nucleus), impacts a myriad of functions ranging from muscle growth and repair to immune function support and libido, to name a few.

Strength training is a well known contributor to increasing testosterone levels. Following a single bout of strength training, testosterone levels rise temporarily and then about an hour later, are reduced.[90] Other research finds that testosterone increases after a single bout of aerobic exercise as well.[93] However, long term aerobic exercise (e.g., marathon) appears to depress testosterone levels.[94]

The time in which testosterone levels remain depressed after resistance training is debatable and probably varies with a number of factors including type of exercise, intensity, volume, etc. The degree of secretion also depends on several factors. For example, compound exercises (e.g., squats, etc.) elicit a greater testosterone surge than do single joint exercises (e.g., biceps curls). It also appears that performing larger muscle exercises first elicits a greater response than performing exercises that use smaller muscle groups first. Also, the resistance used plays a role with heavier resistances (i.e., 5RM to 10 RM) resulting in a greater magnitude of release than lighter resistances. Likewise, performing multiple sets appears superior to single sets. According to some research, at least four sets might be needed to elevate testosterone.[91] The volume of exercise refers to the total amount of weight lifted and is found by calculating sets X reps X resistance used. It appears that testosterone levels elevate more with moderate to high volume exercise.

Exercise Factors Involved In Raising Testosterone Levels

Large muscle exercises	Volume: high to moderate
Heavy resistance (85%-95% 1RM)	Rest: 30 sec to 1 min between sets

In addition there is some evidence that experienced lifter's (> 2 years) may see greater testosterone surges than novice lifter's.[92] This may be at least partially due to experienced lifter's ability to engage in the intense training thought to be required to elicit testosterone elevations.

Alcohol consumption is one factor that has not received a lot of attention in terms of exercise. However, a review of the evidence suggests it can reduce free and bound testosterone in both men and women.[90] In theory, this might upset the testosterone to estrogen ratio and impact muscle and strength development. Based on some evidence, consuming more than 12 oz of beer can reduce testosterone levels in men while up to 12 oz might temporarily raise testosterone levels.[90]

Strength Training and Growth Hormone

Human growth hormone (GH or HG) also called somatotropin is a protein-based hormone secreted from the anterior pituitary gland that acts to strengthen tendons, bones as well as muscles. GH also plays other roles such as immune system support. While generally considered as a single hormone, GH actually represents a family of related compounds that is only now starting to be understood. With respect to resistance training, GH stimulates the usage of amino acids, which contributes to protein synthesis and muscle hypertrophy, while at the same time decreases protein breakdown and speeds up tissue repair. Other effects of GH include decreased use of glucose for fuel while increasing fat usage.

Effects of Growth Hormone

Enhances fat breakdown (lipolysis)	Promotes gluconeogenesis	Possible bone growth stimulation*
Stimulates immune system	Promotes protein anabolism	Possible increased epidermis thickness*
Stimulates cartilage growth	Decreases glycogen synthesis	Possible increase in LBM*

* see reference 96

With respect to strength training, multiple sets utilizing exercises that recruit large muscle groups coupled with heavy loads (e.g., 10 RM) and short rest periods (30 sec - 1 min) appear to be best for significantly elevating GH release.[95] Note that protocols to elevate GH are similar to that required to elevate testosterone. GH levels may remain elevated for 15-30 minutes postexercise.[95]

Much of the effects attributed to GH are actually a result of other compounds called insulin-like growth factors (IGFs) which are secreted by the liver when stimulated by GH. They are called IGF because they resemble the hormone, insulin. The term somatomedin is another name for IGFs. It's important to note that there are several members of the IGF family of compounds.

Sometimes GH is touted as the "fountain of youth." Most claims on this issue stem from a 1990 study of six months of GH injections in older men.[96] This study found that in older men (with low GH levels), GH injections resulted in reduced body fat (14.4%), increased lumbar vertebrae thickness (1.6%) and an increase in skin thickness (7.1%). However, this study involved GH injections which is decidedly different than orally-taken supplements. Many GH-boosting supplements contain the amino acids arginine and ornithine. While large doses of these amino acids may slightly elevate GH in some people, they have never been shown to boost strength or muscle hypertrophy.[38] For a review of the effects and side effects of these and many other supplements, read my book *Nutritional Supplements: What Works and Why* available at www.Joe-cannon.com. Side effects from GH injections include but may not be limited to unhealthy growth of the heart (cardiomyopathy) carpal tunnel syndrome, insulin resistance (which can increase diabetes risk) and unhealthy enlargement of the kidneys and bones.[95]

Growth Hormone: Possible Side Effects

Joint pain	Cardiomyopathy	Increase lean body mass
Carpal tunnel syndrome	Fluid retention	Decreased fat mass
Insulin resistance	Possible increased cancer risk	Elevated blood pressure*

* see reference 96

Cortisol

Cortisol is also called adrenocortical steroid, because it is made in the adrenal glands (located on top of the kidneys) upon stimulation from the hypothalamus gland of the brain. While testosterone is considered an anabolic hormone, cortisol is probably what most fitness people think of when they hear the word catabolic – and for good reason. This hormone facilitates gluconeogenesis, the converting of amino acids and other compounds into glucose. It also inhibits protein synthesis. This serves to increase blood sugar levels during times of fasting. In this respect, cortisol acts similarly to glucagon which also raises blood sugar levels.

Like testosterone, most cortisol in the blood is thought to be bound by proteins (called corticosteroid-binding globulin) as it travels through the body. Only about 10% of the hormone is the free, "active" form. Normally cortisol levels rise quickly in response to a stress, whether it is low blood sugar, surgery or intense exercise. With respect to exercise, avoiding cortisol does not seem to be an option. Studies show that the same types of activities that elicit testosterone and GH release also result in cortisol increases. The good news, however, is that regular exercise appears to reduce the effects of cortisol.[77] This appears to be true in both untrained and exercise-trained individuals.[111] Thus, so called "anti-catabolic" supplements used to reduce cortisol are probably not needed by healthy person's who eat a well balanced diet. Intense exercise training, however, (e.g., triathlon) in the absence of adequate rest and nutrition may result in cortisol and other factors that may overwhelm the body and contributing to overtraining syndrome. High volume, high intensity exercise, coupled with short rest periods appear to augment cortisol more than lower intensity routines. The rest period between sets also appears to impact cortisol with longer rest periods (3 minutes) promoting less of a release than shorter rest periods (1 minute).[102] Ironically, this protocol describes many bodybuilding and fitness programs; however, adequate rest, nutrition and proper design of the exercise program can help reduce any possible deleterious effects of this hormone. As mentioned previously, cortisol is involved with the degradation of muscle tissue. Research finds that fast twitch, type II fibers are more affected by cortisol than slow twitch, type I fibers.[77]

While traditionally thought of as a "bad" hormone, cortisol is intimately involved with growing stronger and plays a critical role in rebuilding of muscle after exercise has occurred. Exercise is a stress and does cause damage to muscle. It's the repair process that allows muscle to grow stronger. While much still needs to be uncovered, cortisol, by taking part in the postexercise inflammation and rebuilding process, helps muscles adapt over time.

Chapter 7

CARDIOVASCULAR PHYSIOLOGY

The cardiovascular system (CV system), is made up of a number of structures that assist with the transportation of oxygen, nutrients, hormones and removal of waste products. The main parts of the cardiovascular system are the heart, blood and blood vessels. The lungs are also included because this is where that the blood gives off its carbon dioxide and is infused with fresh oxygen.

The heart is the pump that is responsible for pushing blood through the CV system. The major blood vessels are called *arteries* and *veins*. A good way to remember each is to keep in mind that, in general, arteries carry oxygen-rich blood *away* from the heart. Veins return oxygen-depleted blood back to the heart. As blood travels further away from the heart, the arteries get smaller and smaller. Smaller arteries are called *arterioles*. These eventually get even smaller and are called *capillaries*. It is in the capillaries that oxygen and other nutrients are exchanged for waste products. On the return trip back to the heart, small blood vessels called *venioles* eventually widen into veins which return blood to the heart.

Blood

The average human adult has about 10 pints of blood in his/her body. Blood is a tissue that consists of a watery portion (plasma) and a cellular portion. Just a few of the cells contained in blood are red blood cells (RBCs) and a host of infection-fighting white blood cells (WBCs). It is the RBCs that carry oxygen throughout the body. Specifically, every red blood cell can carry about 4 oxygen molecules.[22] Red blood cells are able to transport oxygen because they contain an iron-rich compound called hemoglobin which is responsible for giving blood its red color. Red blood cells are made within the bone marrow of bones. An interesting fact about hemoglobin is that as much as it *likes* oxygen, it *loves* carbon monoxide, an odorless, yet toxic gas.[22] This is the reason for successful suicides by those who lock themselves in the garage with the car running. Even in low concentrations carbon monoxide can cause fatigue, chest pain and impair vision and coordination.[23] Cigarettes also contain carbon monoxide and this is one of the reasons that warning labels often mention its presence.

Functions of Blood[*]

• Carries oxygen	• Regulates temperature	• Remove waste products
• Blood clotting	• Regulates pH of blood	• Transports hormones

* Not a complete list

It is blood's ability to carry oxygen that is at the heart of many nutritional and pharmacological attempts to amplify blood volume. Blood doping is a generic term used to describe various ways to boost red blood cell production and enhance exercise performance. For example, one method involves injecting the hormone erythropoietin (EPO) that makes red blood cells. Normally we make EPO when we need RBCs. Some athletes may also use it in the hopes it will give them an advantage in their sport. Blood doping is illegal in many sports including the Olympics because it carries severe side effects, including death.[19] Increased red blood cell concentration means that the blood gets thicker (more viscous). During exercise, water loss via sweat increases the blood's viscosity even more. Eventually, the strain of pumping this gooey mess overwhelms the heart which can result in a heart attack. One natural— and legal— way to enhance red blood cells is by exercising at higher altitudes. Greater altitudes have lower levels of breathable oxygen. After a few weeks, the body compensates by naturally making more red blood cells. It is important to remember however that exercise in general will increase red blood cell production no matter what the altitude.

The Lungs

While usually grouped with the respiratory system, the lungs are also crucial to the functioning of the cardiovascular system because it is here that blood gives up the carbon dioxide (CO_2) that it picked up at the working muscles and is infused with fresh oxygen. Humans have two lungs – a left lung and a right lung. Far from just empty sacs in our chest, the lungs are very complex and have a surface area, which, if stretched out, could cover more than a tennis court.[21] This fantastic surface area is integral to our ability to breathe and continue to live.

Air travels to the lungs via the *trachea*. Each lung is further subdivided into smaller airways called *bronchioles* which eventually lead to small air sacs called *alveoli*. It is here, at the alveoli that the blood receives new oxygen and gives up carbon dioxide gas. Each of the 300 million alveoli that are present in the lungs are surrounded by tiny capillaries which allow for the gas exchange to take place.[39] Gas exchange within the lungs is made possible because of the different concentrations of oxygen and carbon dioxide. In simple terms, things move from where there is a lot of something to where there is less. Since there is more oxygen in the lungs than in the oxygen-depleted RBCs, oxygen enters the RBCs and bonds to hemoglobin. Since there is less CO_2 in the lungs than in the blood, CO_2 leaves the blood and is exhaled from the body. The reverse happens when oxygen-rich blood reaches the cells of your body because the cells have a lot of CO_2 and little oxygen. The other reason this happens is because of what is called the *Bohr Effect*. This refers to the fact that the higher relative acidity of the working muscles weakens the chemical bond between hemoglobin and oxygen. A weaker bond means that oxygen is more likely to leave hemoglobin and go to the cells of the body where it can be used to produce energy.

All humans have areas of the respiratory tract which do not take part in gas exchange. This is referred to as *dead space. Anatomic dead space* includes conducting pathways that do not take part in gas exchange like the trachea and mouth. *Physiologic dead space,* on the other hand, refers to portions of the lungs that do not partake in gas exchange. Fortunately, physiologic dead space is only small part of the lungs.

The control centers of breathing are found in the brain, specifically in a structure called the *medulla* (brain stem). The brain knows when to tell the lungs to inhale and exhale because it has specialized receptors called *chemoreceptors* that monitor the acidity of the blood. Because high levels of CO_2 indicate that the blood is becoming too acidic (i.e., decreased pH), when the brain detects that CO_2 levels are getting too high (or O2 levels get too low) it sends the signal to the lungs to inhale. There are basically two different types of chemoreceptors: *central chemoreceptors* monitor CO_2 levels. *Peripheral chemoreceptors* keep tabs on oxygen levels. While both are important it is the central chemoreceptors that are most important because by keeping track of CO_2 levels, central chemoreceptors also keep tabs on pH levels. Remember, the body does not want to be too acidic as this can affect the overall physiological balance (homeostasis) of the body. Sometimes, when people go diving underwater, they first hyperventilate. When they do this, they breathe faster than they normally do. This lowers the CO_2 levels in their blood and resets the brain's signal to cause you to inhale. In this way you are able to stay underwater for a little longer. Eventually though, the lack of oxygen is detected by your chemoreceptors and you are forced to breath again.

With respect to the lungs, there are some terms to be familiar with. They are:

1. **Tidal Volume:** The tidal volume is the volume of air that can be inhaled or exhaled in a single normal breath.[24] An average young adult inhales and exhales about a pint (500 ml) of air with each breath.[24]
2. **Vital Capacity:** The maximum volume of air that can be exhaled after the person has inhaled as much as they can.[24] In a young adult this equals about a gallon of air (4600 ml).[24]
3. **Residual Volume.** Even after a person has exhaled as much as he/she can, some air will remain in the lungs. This is the residual volume. For an adult, this usually averages about 2 pints (1200 ml).[24]

These terms (especially the first two) are sometimes measured medically in athletes so you may run into them one day.

Basic Anatomy of the Heart

Of all the muscles of the body, the heart is undoubtedly the most important. This organ, about the size of a fist, contracts (beats) an average of 100,000 time a day and pumps about 2,000 gallons of blood each day![18] For those who live until the age of 80, the heart has performed at least 2.9 billion beats![41] The human heart has four chambers: 2 *atria* and 2 *ventricles*. Between the atria and ventricles are a series of valves (flaps of connective tissue). These valves make sure that blood only travels in one direction. The valve between the right atria and right ventricle is called the *tricuspid valve*. The valve between the left atria and left ventricle is called the *bicuspid valve* (or mitral valve). The heart walls themselves are made up of three distinct layers: the outer *epicardium* layer, a middle layer called the *myocardium* and an inner layer called the *endocardium*.

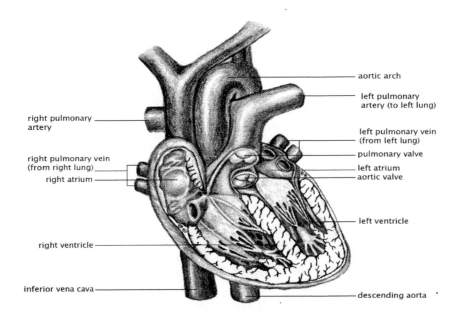

Heart Muscle vs. Skeletal Muscle

Both heart muscle and skeletal muscle are similar in that they both are striated, containing actin and myosin muscle proteins. They also both contract according to the sliding filament theory. They differ, however, in a few key areas. For one, heart muscle has the ability to contract on its own. This is a very good thing since nobody wants to keep remembering to tell their heart to beat! Another difference is that there is just one type of heart muscle rather than different types of skeletal muscle (slow twitch and fast twitch). Specifically, heart muscle is very aerobic in nature, possessing many similarities to that of slow twitch, type I fibers found in skeletal muscles. Another important difference is that heart muscle cells are connected to each other by way of what are called *intercalated disks*. The word, intercalate, means to insert between something. Intercalated disks are inserted between heart cells and allow for the speedy transmission of nerve impulses from one heart cell to another. It is because of intercalated disks that the heart is able to contract as a single unit.

The heart is furnished with its own blood supply via the *left and right coronary arteries* which supply blood to the left and right sides of the heart respectively. The coronary arteries begin as branching off points of the aorta and then further spread out over the heat to ensure adequate distribution of oxygen and nutrients throughout the myocardium. Blood leaves the heart by way of the coronary veins. For those who have trouble remembering which is which, remember as a rule, arteries contain high levels of oxygen and nutrients while veins contain low levels.

The path that blood takes through the heart is as follows: Blood enters the heart via two large veins – the *superior vena cava* and *inferior vena cava*. Both of these veins empty into the right atrium of the heart. From the right atrium, blood then travels to the right ventricle. From there, blood passes into the lungs via the pulmonary arteries where blood gives off its carbon dioxide and is infused with fresh oxygen. After this, blood leaves the lungs and passes into the left atrium and finally into the left ventricle. It is from the left ventricle that blood is ejected from the heart and travels to all parts of the body. Eventually, blood that is low in oxygen and nutrients returns to the heart again via superior and inferior vena cava. This return of oxygen-poor blood to the heart is called *venous return*.

The heart muscle surrounding the left ventricle is thicker than at other areas of the heart. This makes sense because the force created by the contracting left ventricle is what propels the blood out of the heart. It is interesting to note that with exercise training, this left ventricular heart muscle actually gets stronger. A stronger left ventricle means that one can eject more blood out of the heart in a given moment of time. This is an example of one of the positive changes that occur in the body when one undertakes an exercise program.

When blood leaves the heart it does so through its main artery – the aorta. The aorta, as it travels up the sides of the neck, branches off (forks) and goes in different directions. The point at which the aorta branches off is subjected to high pressures as blood coerces through the circulatory system. Over time – especially with hypertension – this branch point can be a cause of concern on the part of physicians because it is an area that can develop artery-clogging plaque. In extreme cases surgery may be needed to correct this problem.

Some may wonder how the heart contracts. In other words, what is the driving force that compels the heart to beat? The heart contracts when an electrical signal spreads through the heart in an orderly fashion. As a portion of the heart encounters the electoral impulse, that section contracts.

The electrical signal that is responsible for the heartbeat originates within the heart itself, in an area of the right atrium called the *sinoatrial node* (SA node). The SA node is sometimes called the "pacemaker" because it has the fastest rate (usually 60-100 bpm) of contraction and sets the pace that the rest of the heart follows. When the signal spreads outward from the SA node it soon encounters an area called the *atrioventricular node* (AV node) which is also found in the right atrium. The AV node is what allows the electrical signal to pass through the heart's chambers in an orderly fashion and prevents the chambers from contracting at the same time. More specifically, when the electrical signal encounters the AV node, its speed slows down and is redirected through the various nerve fibers that spread out over the ventricles (these are called *left and right bundle branches*, sometimes called the *Bundle of His*). These then lead to other pathways called *Purkinje fibers* that further transmit the electrical signal over the ventricles. In this way, the electoral signal is conducted in such a way that the heart beats in a uniform fashion.

Impulse Signal Pathway within the Heart

The electrical signal that stimulates heart contraction takes this path:

1. SA node starts the signal. The signal then travels to:
2. The AV node. From there the signal goes to:
3. Left and right bundle branches. Then it goes to:
4. Purkinje fibers. From the Purkinje fibers the signal makes contact with individual heart cells called "cardiocytes."

Blood Flow to the Organs

While all organs receive blood, the flow of the blood to various organs is restricted under some circumstances (like exercise, for example). But, how does the blood know where to go? Basically, blood goes to where it's needed most. This is accomplished by a complex interaction between the blood vessels, the nervous system and various chemical messengers that all work together. For example, with exercise, a large percentage of the blood is directed to the exercising muscles. In this instance, less blood goes to the digestive system. Both the parasympathetic and sympathetic divisions of the nervous system send signals that expand and constrict blood vessels. Some of these impulses cause blood vessels to constrict (called *vasoconstriction*) which increases the resistance to blood flow. Other impulses cause blood vessels to expand (called *vasodilatation*). This increases blood flow to an area. Some reading these words may be familiar with the amino acid arginine which is metabolized to a gas called nitric oxide (NO). Nitric oxide is a potent vasodilator that might help improve some symptoms of heart disease in older individuals.[37] Because of its vasodilatory effects, some fitness enthusiasts may experiment with arginine/"NO supplements" in the hopes of speeding recovery, improving strength or enhancing the "pumped" look of muscles following exercise. Most of these claims, though, needs more study.[38] Conversely, compounds that act as vasoconstrictors include thromboxane and epinephrine (adrenalin).

So how does the brain "know" when blood pressure changes? *Baroreceptors* are specialized pressure receptors within blood vessels which monitor blood pressure changes and relay the information to the brain. Baroreceptors are found in the aortic arch of the aorta as well as in the carotid arteries. They are sensitive to blood pressure changes and constantly relay information back to the brain.

Measuring Pulse

In the past, you may have measured your pulse by lightly feeling the carotid artery on the side of your neck. While this may work fine for you, it is usually not appropriate for other people. If you press too hard on the neck, you activate the baroreceptors in the carotid artery which, *reduce* heart rate. This will result in an inaccurate measurement of a person's resting heart rate (RHR). For better results, measure RHR at the *radial pulse* which is located on the thumb side of the wrist.

Blood Pressure and the Heart

Blood pressure and the heart are intimately related. In fact, blood pressure is the result of the heart pumping blood through the blood vessels. When the heart beats, it pushes blood out of the heart. This results in what is called the *systolic blood pressure*. When the heart fills with blood, before it contracts again, this results in the *diastolic pressure*. So, the blood pressure that you measure is the combination of two separate pressures – systolic and diastolic blood pressures. These are written as a fraction. The systolic is the top number of the fraction and the diastolic pressure is the bottom number. For example, if your blood pressure was 122/75, the systolic BP is 122 and 75 is the diastolic BP.

With aerobic exercise, the systolic BP tends to increase as exercise intensity is ramped up. The diastolic BP, on the other hand, usually remains constant or decreases a point or so. For example, the increase in BP might look like this: 120/80, 135/80, 150/80 and so on. With respect to resistance (strength) training, both systolic and diastolic blood pressure can increase dramatically, especially if combined with the Valsalva effect. In fact, blood pressures greater than 355/281 have been measured with strength training! However BP tends to return to normal shortly after cessation of exercise or before the next set is preformed.[74]

When working with clients who have heart, kidney or blood pressure issues, it is prudent to measure blood pressure before and after exercise. This can tell you not only how the exercise program you designed is affecting them but also can give you valuable information on whether or not they should exercise to begin with. Specifically, people whose resting blood pressure is ≥ 200/115 mmHg or close to this amount, should not exercise.[1] Rather, they should be referred back to their physician who can then take the appropriate action.

Blood Pressure Guidelines[75]

<120/80	Normal
120/80 -139/89	Prehypertension
≥140/90	Hypertension

Notice that blood pressures of 120/80 are not called "normal" any longer. Technically less than 120/80 is normal. A BP of 120/80 is now referred to as "prehypertension" or pre high blood pressure. This change was made in light of evidence finding that in men, age 55 years, who started out with a BP of 120/80 appear to have a 90% chance of developing high blood pressure at some point in their lives.[75] So, is 120/80 "normal" or is it really a prelude to high blood pressure?

Everyone should know his/her blood pressure. Hypertension can lead to stroke – the 3rd leading cause of death in the US!

Rate Pressure Product

The *rate pressure product*, also called, *double product* is equal to the heart rate multiplied by the systolic blood pressure and is a factor used by medical professionals to estimate how much oxygen the heart is using. In other words, it measures how hard the heart is working. When either heart rate or systolic blood pressure (or both) is elevated (as with exercise), the heart works harder. In healthy people who exercise regularly, rate pressure product is generally lower because exercise can lower resting heart rate and/or systolic blood pressure. Thus, when taken at rest, a lower rate pressure product usually means that the exercise-trained heart does not have to work as hard.

Heart Attack Warning Signs[156]

Constant or intermittent discomfort in the middle of the chest*	Shortness of breath*	Breaking out in cold sweats
Jaw pain*	Nausea and/or vomiting*	Back pain*
Neck pain	Lightheadedness	Pain in one or both arms

* Common warning signs in women

Stroke Warning Signs[156]

Numbness or weakness in face, arm or leg, particularly on one side of the body only	Sudden confusion or trouble speaking or understanding	Sudden trouble seeing in one or both eyes
Sudden trouble walking	Sudden loss of balance/coordination	Sudden headache with no known cause

How the Nervous System Affects Heart Rate

If the SA node usually sets the rhythm of the heart by beating between 60-100 bpm, how is it possible that people can have heart rates lower and higher than this? For example, depending on the age of the person, during exercise it's possible to have heart rates of 150 bpm or more! This is where the nervous system comes into play.

The *central nervous system* (CNS) consists of the brain and spinal cord. An extension of the CNS is the *peripheral nervous system* (PNS). The peripheral nervous system includes the nerves that stimulate organ systems outside of the brain and spinal cord, like arms, legs, abdominals and even the heart.

The PNS can be divided into two parts: the *sympathetic nervous system* and the *parasympathetic nervous system*. This may sound confusing but in reality it's not. The sympathetic nervous system is what speeds up the heart rate. The parasympathetic nervous system slows the heart rate down. This is why it's possible to have heart rates above and below the rate dictated by the SA node. Looking at this another way, think of them like your car's accelerator pedal. When you press down on the accelerator, the car goes faster. This is what the sympathetic nervous system does. When you take your foot off the accelerator, the car slows down. This is like the parasympathetic nervous system.

It is well known that people who exercise regularly have lower resting heart rates than non-exercisers. The reason for this is because of the parasympathetic nervous system. In those who work out regularly, the parasympathetic nervous system exerts greater control over the heart rate, causing RHR to decrease.

Sympathetic vs. Parasympathetic Nervous System [*]

Sympathetic Nervous System	Parasympathetic Nervous System
Mobilizes energy in times of stress	Control of Sex
Increases heart rate	Conserves energy during times of rest
Increases force of muscle contractions	Decreases blood pressure
Reroutes blood to working muscles, away from digestive system	Decreases breathing rate
Increases glucose levels in blood	Stimulates digestion

*Not a complete list

How Well Is Your Heart Pumping?

The heart plays a major role in how well we can exercise. While the interaction of the heart with exercise is complex, personal trainers should be familiar with a few heart-related concepts so that that they can interact intelligently with other health professionals and better explain to their clients some of the changes that occur when one undertakes a regular exercise program.

One of the factors relating to the heart is the *stroke volume* (SV), which is the amount of blood pumped out of the heart (specifically, from the left ventricle) per heart beat. Each time the heart beats, it ejects some blood. That amount is simply called the stroke volume. Technically, the stroke volume is also defined by the equation SV = EDV – ESV. End systolic volume (ESV) is the volume of blood in the heart after it has contracted (systole). End diastolic volume (EDV) is the amount of blood contained inside the left ventricle at the end of its filling phase (diastole). Another way of saying this is that EDV is the amount of blood in the heart just before it contracts. This gives rise to the other name for EDV —"preload." In other words, it's the amount of blood that the heart is "loaded" with before it contracts. As preload increases, stroke volume also increases.

Just as air stretches a balloon when you inflate it, the volume of blood inside the heart prior to contraction also exerts a stretching force on the heart walls. The greater the volume of blood in the heart means the greater the stretch force – and also the greater the recoil force as the heart contracts. This rubber-band recoil-like effect of the heart adds to its ability to eject blood and is referred to as the *Frank-Starling Law of the Heart*, named in honor of the two scientists who first described this effect. In essence, this law says that the more blood that fills the heart before it contracts, results in a greater volume of blood that is ejected from the heart. This, in turn, allows each heartbeat to deliver more blood to the cardiovascular system and is another reason why we are able to exercise at higher intensities. Remember *preload* described above? Well, exercise professionals may also discuss *afterload*. Afterload describes how hard it is to eject blood from the heart. In order for blood to leave the heart, the pressure of the blood in the left ventricle must be greater than the overall blood pressure. If the pressure outside the heart is greater than that inside the heart, less blood is ejected. This reduces not only cardiac output and stroke volume but overall health as well.

High blood pressure (hypertension) is a condition that can increase afterload. Holding breath during weight lifting (Valsalva maneuver) also increases afterload and can lead to one losing consciousness.

End systolic volume (ESV) is the amount of blood in the heart just after the heart contracts (some blood will remain inside the left ventricle after each contraction). An increased stroke volume means the heart is getting more efficient by pumping more blood with each heart beat. This is another factor that contributes to a slower heart rate in exercise-trained individuals.

Another heart-function term is called the *ejection fraction*. As stated previously, some blood remains inside the left ventricle after the heart contracts. This is normal. If we could measure the amount of blood within the left ventricle before it contracted (the end diastolic volume) and compare that to the amount that was ejected (stroke volume), we would get a fraction – the ejection fraction! Another way of saying this is that the ejection fraction is the percent of the blood that is actually ejected from the left ventricle of the heart compared to what was in the left ventricle before it contracted. Normally, the heart ejects about 2/3 (67%) of left ventricular volume with each heartbeat. Exercise-trained hearts have even greater ejection fractions In fact, in highly trained athletes ejection fraction might be more than 90%! In people who have heart disease, ejection might be only 20%. Mathematically, ejection fraction can be calculated from two different-looking, yet identical equations:

$$EF = SV/EDV \quad \text{and} \quad EF = \frac{EDV - ESV}{EDV}$$

Where EF is ejection fraction, SV is stroke volume, EDV is end diastolic volume and ESV is end systolic volume.

The third heart-related term is called the *cardiac output* (sometimes abbreviated as CO or Q). Cardiac output is the amount of blood pumped from the heart (specifically, from the left ventricle) in one minute. Cardiac output is found by multiplying the heart rate times the stroke volume. This gives rise to the classic equation used to describe cardiac output: CO = HR X SV. Thus, as heart rate and stroke volume increase, cardiac output also increases. During exercise in an upright position like running, walking or cycling, cardiac output increases because both stroke volume and heart rate increase.[29] Like the other two values described above – stroke volume and ejection fraction – those who exercise on a regular basis tend to have greater cardiac outputs than non-exercisers.

Obviously, fitness trainers will probably not be calculating stroke volumes, ejection fractions or cardiac outputs. The equations are presented here to help give you a better understanding of these concepts and help you explain them to clients if the need arises. In addition, sometimes fitness professionals may find themselves interacting with other members of the health care continuum like physicians, chiropractors and nurses, to name a few. Knowledge of these and other concepts discussed in this book goes a long way in establishing yourself as a competent member of their team.

Blood Flow During Exercise

Blood is the source of oxygen and nutrients. This means blood is a valuable currency. Just as you might allocate your money to pay different bills, so, too, does the body. During exercise, the body automatically redistributes blood flow such that the muscles and organ systems that are participating in exercise get the most blood while those muscles and organ systems that are not, receive a reduced blood flow. For example, during maximal exercise up to 75%-90% of cardiac output is shunted toward the working muscles compared to only 15% -20% at rest.[29]

Acute Changes from CV Exercise

Acute changes refer to short term changes that occur soon after exercise begins. In other words, after you're working out for a few seconds to many minutes. Before you even enter the gym or step on a treadmill, your heart rate will begin to increase. This is the body's way of preparing itself for exercise. Related to this, stroke volume, ejection fraction and cardiac output also increase during exercise.

As you exercise, one of the first changes occurs within the blood vessels just under the skin: a vasodilation (opening up) of blood vessels occurs, allowing blood to come close to the skin's surface and give off excess heat. In this way, the body helps to cool itself during exercise.

Blood flow to the muscles changes also. Specifically, muscle blood flow tends to be about 15%-20% of cardiac output at rest but with exercise may increase to as much as 75% for most people and as much as 90% in some elite athletes![41] This occurs because blood goes to where it is needed most. Conversely, blood flow to other organ systems decreases. For example, blood flow to the stomach and other digestive systems is usually reduced during exercise.

As for blood pressure during exercise, remember that systolic blood pressure tends to increase as exercise intensity increases. Diastolic blood pressure, on the other hand, either tends to remain constant or may decrease a little.

Various hormones also begin to change with exercise. As you exercise, your cells are using glucose (sugar) to help power your exercising muscles. *Glucagon* is a hormone that's made in the pancreas, which raises blood sugar. Glucagon begins to increase during exercise. With respect to insulin, it tends to be reduced during exercise. This may seem backward to some because insulin, which is also made in the pancreas, is needed in order for sugar (glucose) to be used by the cells of the body. However, even though less insulin is released, the body, during exercise, is more efficient at using insulin. Also when we exercise, we ramp up the use of non-insulin dependant sugar gateways. These gateways do not need insulin to work. Thus, by becoming more efficient at using insulin and activating alternate pathways for glucose to enter the cells, the body doesn't need as much insulin during exercise. As you might guess, this has important implications for diabetics as well.

Epinephrine (adrenaline) made in the adrenal glands is another hormone which helps boost glucose levels and heart rate. It also increases overall alertness and assists with fat metabolism. Epinephrine tends to increase during exercise and also produces more forceful muscle contractions.

Growth hormone (GH) increases during exercise, especially in untrained person's. Growth hormone impacts a range of body systems including immune function and muscle growth. As a rule, resistance training is superior to endurance exercise at increasing GH levels.

Summary: Effects of an Acute bout of Aerobic Exercise[*]

Parameter	Exercise Effect
Heart rate	Increases before exercise begins. Increases also as exercise intensity increases.
Stroke volume, ejection fraction, cardiac output	All increase with increasing exercise intensities.
Blood flow to skin	Increases to help dissipate heat; blood flow to working muscles increases; decreased flow to "non-priority" organ systems.
Blood pressure	Systolic increases; diastolic remains constant or decreases slightly.

Glucagon	Increases
Insulin	Decreases. Cell sensitivity to insulin increases.
Epinephrine	Increases
Growth hormone	Increases

* Not a complete list

Chronic Adaptations from CV Exercise

Chronic (long term) aerobic exercise results in several changes (adaptations) of the heart and overall cardiovascular system as well as to other body systems. Fitness trainers should have a working knowledge of how chronic exercise changes the body so that they can best develop effective exercise programs for their clients. Below are just a few of the positive adaptations associated with long-term aerobic exercise.

Probably one of the most dramatic changes that has been observed is that almost across the board, the risk from dying tends to decrease in person's who exercise on a regular basis.[1] The amount of exercise thought to be sufficient for this purpose varies from expert to expert but is generally 30-60 minutes performed most days of the week.

Many fitness trainers are aware that the resting heart rate decreases following exercise training. This effect may be observed in as few as two weeks of training but may take as many as ten weeks or more in some cases.[27] As mentioned previously, this decrease in RHR is thought to be the result of an increase in parasympathetic nervous activity coupled with a decrease in the influence of sympathetic nervous system. In addition, heart rate during exercise also is reduced. Specifically, heart rate during submaximal exercise (less than an all-out effort) is lower than that of someone not used to exercise. This happens because with exercise training the heart gets stronger. Thus, what would have over-stressed the heart before, no longer does.

With respect to the heart itself, we see that it enlarges from long-term exercise. This makes sense because just as a muscle grows in size when it's exercised, so too does the heart. Specifically, not only do the chambers of the heart increase but also the thickness of the heart muscle itself. This is especially true for the muscle of the left ventricle.[42]

After exercise, the heart rate does not immediately return to normal. Rather, a little time is needed and this is sometimes referred to as the heart rate recovery period. In people who are more fit, the heart rate returns to normal faster.[42]

Regular aerobic exercise stimulates the body to ramp up its blood production. Specifically, not only are more red blood cells (and hemoglobin) made but the watery, fluid part of blood (plasma) also increases. This increase in blood volume means more blood enters and leaves the heart with each beat.

Capillaries are the smallest blood vessels in the body and it is here that oxygen and nutrients pass from the blood into the cells. Long-term aerobic exercise results in an increase in capillaries and this increase is greatest with respect to the muscles that are actively participating in the exercise.[28] In other words, if you were a runner, we'd expect to see increased capillary density in the legs. Other research suggests that the capillaries within the heart itself also increase following aerobic endurance exercise.[43] This suggests that the heart may be better at absorbing oxygen and nutrients!

In some studies blood pressure has been shown to decrease following long term aerobic exercise.[1] Specifically, both systolic and diastolic blood pressure might lower following exercise training.[30] This effect seems to be greatest in people with hypertension as opposed to those with more normal blood pressures.[30]

Scientists can estimate which macronutrient (fat, carbohydrate or protein) your body is primarily using (burning) by measuring the amounts (ratio) of oxygen and carbon dioxide that you inhale and exhale. This gives rise to the *respiratory exchange ratio* (RER). Mathematically, RER is equal to the volume of carbon dioxide exhaled divided by the volume of oxygen inhaled.[42] Another way of saying this is that RER = VCO2 / VO2. Mathematics aside, an RER of 1.00 means you are burning all of your energy from carbohydrates; an RER of about 0.7 means you are burring all of your energy from fat. An RER of about 0.82 means you're burning all protein. At rest our RER is somewhere between 0.7 and 1.0, meaning we are burning a mixture of fats and carbohydrates. In fact, we tend to burn a little more fat than carbs at rest (remember, we burn a greater percentage of fat during low intensity, long duration activities – including rest). It turns out that after several months of exercise training, RER decreases during exercise at submaximal levels (i.e., it moves closer to 0.7). This means that exercise-trained people burn fat better than those who don't exercise regularly. As a personal trainer it is unlikely that you ever calculate RER. However, remembering the RER numbers can be valuable if your career path leads you to working with athletes, weight loss or advanced exercise testing.

Many studies also find that exercise (especially aerobic exercise) produces favorable changes in total cholesterol as well as HDL and LDL. More to the point, exercise has been shown to reduce total cholesterol and LDL ("bad" cholesterol) as well as raise HDL ("good" cholesterol).[30,31] Levels of triglycerides have also been shown to reduce following exercise training.[30] These results have been in observed in both men and women. This, of course, tends to reduce the incidence of coronary artery disease (CAD), also known as heart disease, which is the number one killer of Americans. It is noteworthy to mention that while the usual recommendations call for at least 30 minutes of continuous aerobic exercise on most days of the week, some research also suggests that splitting exercise into smaller blocks of time also appears to promote health benefits in ways similar to that of continuous exercise.[32,33] This is useful information for people with busy schedules who often complain that they do not have time to exercise.

Studies show the moderate levels of exercise training can help improve various aspects of the immune system.[45] Exhaustive exercise (i.e., running a marathon), however, is associated with decreased immunity.[44]

Lastly, one often-neglected adaptation involves the body's own antioxidant defense systems. Remember that antioxidants neutralize potentially damaging compounds called *free radicals*. Many people may be under the assumption that antioxidants can only be obtained from nutritional supplements (e.g., vitamin C and vitamin E). They are unaware that the body has an array of internal antioxidant defenses that help protect us from free radicals. These defenses include enzymes like *superoxide dismutase* (SOD for short), *catalase* and *glutathione peroxidase*. Studies indicate that exercise training can result in an increase in many of these enzymes and probably other defenses as well.[34]

Summary: Effects of Long Term Aerobic Exercise*

Parameter	How Exercise Helps
Death from all causes	Risk decreases
Resting heart rate	Tends to lower
Submaximal exercise heart rate	Tends to lower
Overall heart size	Tends to enlarge somewhat
Muscles of left ventricle	Tend to enlarge and grow stronger

Blood	Increase in RBCs, hemoglobin and plasma
Stroke volume, ejection fraction and cardiac output	All tend to increase
Capillary density of working muscles	Tends to increase
Heart capillary density	Tends to increase
Blood pressure	Both systolic & diastolic tend to lower – especially in those with high blood pressure
Cholesterol, LDL & triglycerides	Tends to be reduced
Ability to burn fat (RER)	Greater ability to burn fat
HDL	Tends to increase
Immunity	Improved with moderate levels of exercise
Body's antioxidant defense systems	Tends to increase

* Not a complete list

It is important to keep in mind that everybody is different and not everyone will experience the same results from chronic aerobic conditioning. For example, you might expect a sedentary individual to have a greater magnitude of a response compared to an athlete. Also, if physical activity is not continued on a regular basis, strength and endurance may begin to diminish after about 2-3 weeks. For highly trained individuals who are close to their full genetic potential, some loss may occur after less than a week. Other factors may take longer or lesser time before they revert to pre-exercise conditions.

Chapter 8

DESIGNING EXERCISE PROGRAMS

This chapter will review many of the basic and essential tools and concepts fitness trainers need to be familiar with when designing an exercise program. While not specifically covered in this chapter, it should be understood that, ideally, before any exercise program can be developed, the client should first undergo some form of fitness testing or interview process to determine weak/strong areas as well as complete the necessary paperwork to enable the trainer to gauge the health and training experience of the individual.

Principles of Training

The following are principles or laws of exercise and are important to be familiar with as they will help guide whatever decisions you may make with regard to putting together an exercise program for a client or yourself.

Principle of Individual Differences

This principle takes into account our innate genetic differences and basically says that each person will respond differently to an exercise program. For example, following the strength training program of the world's strongest man (or woman) may not produce the same results in you if you are not blessed with their genetic abilities.

Principle of Specificity

This principle basically says that a training program should usually progress from very general to very specific exercises. For beginners, an overall basic program that is not very specific is best; then, as fitness improves, it's possible to better target exercise to meet their individual needs and goals. Another definition for this principle states that if your goal is to be better at some specific task, then you have to do that task if it is to improve. This gives rise to the phrase *specific adaptations to imposed demands* (i.e. SAID Principle). While this may sound difficult to understand, it's not. Basically, it means that if you want to be a better runner, then run! If you want to be better at the bench press, do the bench press. The body will respond specifically to those exercise demands that are imposed upon it. To illustrate, I once met with an 80-year old woman who told me that she could lift 130 lbs on the seated leg press, yet when she accidentally slipped and fell, she discovered she was unable to get up from the floor! She wasn't hurt from the fall, but was just not strong enough. This made perfect sense because the leg press, while working many of the same muscles that she would use when rising from the floor, is not the same thing as actually getting up from the floor. After a few weeks of practice, she was able to get up from the floor unassisted!

Principle of Overload

This principle states that no positive change occurs unless the body is overloaded a little more than it is used to. For example, if you could lift 100 lbs 10 times (i.e., you're 10 RM) and you wanted to be stronger, increase the load lifted to 105 lbs. You may not be able to lift it 10 times at first but eventually you will.

We overload the body by basically manipulating one or more of four factors that are collectively called the *FITT Principle*. In essence, the FITT Principle is what makes up the overload principle. The FITT Principe is stands for:

> **Frequency of exercise**. For example, increasing exercise from 2 days a week to 3 days a week.
> **Intensity of exercise**. For example, increasing the weight lifted from 100 lbs to 105 lbs or ramping up the speed on the treadmill from 3 mph to 3.2 mph.
> **Time of exercise**. For example, you might increase your time in the gym from 30 minutes to 40 minutes. If you ever deal with a person who has a special need like someone who has high blood pressure, remember increasing the time of exercise is usually safer than increasing the intensity of exercise.
> **Type of exercise**. An example of this progression would be moving from strength training machines to free weights. Cardio vs. strength training are also different types of activity.

Principle of Progression

This is sometimes called the *principle of progressive overload* and is basically the same as the principle of overload described previously. It refers to exposing the body to new overloads that it can cope with to foster further gains in fitness. With respect to weight lifting, one usually manipulates sets, reps, weight and volume when progressing an individual.

Principle of Maintenance

According to this principle, once you are at the fitness level you're happy with, continue to train at that level to maintain what you have.

Principle of Adaptation

There is a saying in exercise that goes like this: all exercise programs will work – but only for so long. Eventually the body will adapt (get used to) the exercise stimulus and if your goal is to progress, you will have to vary the routine somehow (by altering the FITT Principle).

Principle of Disuse or Reversibility

This is basically the *use it or lose it* principle. If you don't continue to exercise, you'll eventually lose all the benefits you obtained from it in the first place. Depending on one's level of fitness, it's possible to begin to lose fitness after 2 weeks of not training.

Warm Up

Generally, a warm up consists of 5-10 minutes of light aerobic activity. Calisthenics can also be used if they are of sufficient length. The goal of the warm up is to prepare the body for the exercise program. This is sometimes referred to as a *general warm up*. The benefits of warming up are many and include:[1]

1. increased metabolic rate above resting levels
2. improved reaction time
3. improved flexibility
4. possible reduced risk of injury during exercise
5. possible reductions in heart rhythm abnormalities (e.g., heart attack)

In contrast to a general warm up, one may also choose to perform an exercise-specific warm up. For example, performing a few sets of a bench press at a low resistance prior to going heavy would be a more specific warm up. For safety reasons, it's best to always perform a general warm up prior to doing an exercise-specific warm up. It is also important to note that stretching usually does not constitute a good warm up. This is because most people do not stretch long enough.

Stretching and Injuries

Contrary to popular belief, the act of stretching just prior to exercise does not appear to significantly reduce the frequency of sports-related injuries.[103] However, some research suggests that regular stretching may offer a mild protective effect.[104] Likewise, stretching prior to exercise does not appear to significantly reduce delayed onset muscle soreness (DOMS).[103,104] Despite the research, those who take part in ballistic exercise (basketball, etc.) may still want to stretch prior to activity because of the forceful nature of those events.

Classifying types of Exercises

While it may not be immediately apparent, personal trainers, usually make a distinction between exercises on the basis of how much muscle they recruit. This leads to the classifications called multi-joint and single-joint exercises. A *multi-joint exercise* is one which enlists large muscle groups. Squats, bench presses and push ups are examples of multi-joint exercises. Multi-joint exercises are also sometimes called *core exercises* because they should form the basis or core of a strength training program. Another term also used is *compound exercise*. Compound refers to the fact that multi-joint movements result from the interaction of a number of muscle groups. In contrast, a *single-joint exercise* is one that uses less muscle. Biceps curls and triceps extensions are examples of this. While both types of exercises are essential, those that are multi-joint are usually seen as being more important because they tend to be more sports-specific and better mimic one's ADLs.

Another way to classify exercises is to use the terms *open chain* and *closed chain*. Consider a chain you may wear around your neck. If the chain is broken, the ends are free to dangle. An open chain exercise is one in which the feet (or hands) are freely moving (e.g., leg extension). In contrast, a closed chain exercise is one in which the feet (or hands) are stabilized on the floor or other surface and do not move (e.g., leg press). One can think of closed chain as being somewhat similar to multi-joint movements while open chain are somewhat analogous to single-joint movements.

The Order of Exercises: What Comes First, Last, etc.

There is an old saying that goes like this: *Everything works for a little while*. Even the worst designed exercise program will probably work for about a month or two. After that it's probably a good idea to alter the program to foster further improvements. With that in mind, let's review some logical rules to remember when designing a program. Of course there are exceptions to almost every rule; however, following these basic guidelines will help you when you design a program for your clients.

- ➤ **Warm up should occur first.** The warm up can help reduce injury. Never overlook warming up.
- ➤ **Large muscle groups before small muscle groups.** In general, work the chest, back and legs, before biceps, triceps, etc. Multi-joint exercises usually come before single-joint movements. Working the smaller muscles first to "pre-exhaust" them is an advanced technique that should be reserved only for advanced lifter's.
- ➤ **Don't train the same muscles two days in a row.** Remember, muscles grow stronger after exercise. Training the same muscle without enough rest may decrease the benefits and increase injury. Generally, 24-48 hours is recommended between strength training sessions. Depending on the fitness level, difficulty of the routine and age of the individual, even more time may be required.
- ➤ **Power movements should be placed early in the workout.** It's very difficult to exert maximal power so it's safer to do it when the client is strongest. Don't wait until the end of the workout when they are tired.
- ➤ **Skill/agility-related movements should be placed early in workout.** Movements that require balance or a special skill or dexterity should be performed early. Again, put the hardest stuff at the beginning. Depending on the fitness level of the individual, even walking could be considered a skill/agility related movement.
- ➤ **Work abs/low back *after* working muscle groups that involve the abs or low back.** This is important because fatiguing the abs or low back first can reduce their ability to help stabilize the trunk during multi-joint activities. This might increase injury risk. This is usually why people train abs and low back toward the end of the workout.
- ➤ **Work the muscles you want to emphasize the most early in the workout.** Suppose you want to focus on the shoulders. Because you are strongest at the start of the workout, movements that emphasize shoulders in this example would be some of the first muscles targeted.
- ➤ **Perform new exercises early.** Any new activities that you teach a client should be placed early in the workout. This might help reduce injury because the person is strongest and most alert in the beginning.
- ➤ **Progress from machines to free weights.** Machines are usually easier to use, so starting a client with this may be safer. Also, progressing to free weights is not always the goal. Some people may be perfectly happy using machines forever. Keep in mind that some people may be intimidated by free weights.
- ➤ **Do free weights *before* machines – if both are performed in the same workout.** Because machines are usually easier, leaving them until last, in theory, reduces injury while still letting the muscle group be worked. This is an advanced technique.
- ➤ **Cool down.** This is the reversal of the warm up. Cooling down returns the body to its pre-exercise state, can prevent dizziness after exercise and may even help stabilize heart function.[1]

> **Stretch.** Stretching after the workout may be more efficient than stretching before and after exercise, and appears to confer the same benefits.[183]

Abs Everyday?

This question about training abs every day or every other day is hotly debated among fitness trainers. The rationale for working abs every day usually stems from the high concentration of slow twitch, type I fibers found in the abdominal area. These fibers are geared toward endurance and recover faster. Those who say that every other day is best usually base their argument on the fact that during a crunch/sit-up, one is lifting about 50-60% of their body weight. This is somewhat analogous to lifting weights and the guideline for that is usually every other day. So who is right? Both arguments have merit; however, consider the client and his/her fitness level. Unfit people/novices are best served by every other day as this will reduce DOMS and injuries. For more fit people, every day may be ok but to be safe, try different types of ab exercises that work not only the rectus abdominis but the other muscles of the abs. Keep in mind, also that ab exercises alone won't create a "six-pack." That comes from good genetics, aerobic exercise and eating fewer calories.

Designing a Strength Training Program

All exercise programs (strength or cardio) can be said to have the following stages: initial conditioning stage; improvement stage and maintenance stage.

The *initial conditioning stage* is the point in the program when the body first becomes accustomed to the rigors of regular exercise. During this phase a primary goal should be to establish a foundation on which to base future, more difficult training sessions. Other goals should be to bolster confidence, improve muscle endurance, foster a healthy lifestyle and develop a love for working out. Now is not the time to overwhelm someone with multiple sets or produce large degrees of muscle soreness (DOMS). Depending on fitness level, this stage may last for 4-8 weeks and possibly up to 12 weeks.

The *improvement stage* occurs after the initial conditioning stage and is when the exercise stimulus is gradually increased to foster further improvements. Resistances used, as well as intensity of aerobic activity is ramped up – again, according to the client's individual needs, wants and health history. This stage might last for 4-6 months.

At some people the client reaches a point where he/she is happy and doesn't need to progress any further. This *maintenance stage* is where the client basically maintains the fitness level he/she developed up to this point. Doing the same thing all the time can be boring, so this may also be a good time to establish new, attainable goals.

When putting together a strength training program, it is important to have an idea of the basic principles behind achieving various goals. For example, someone desiring muscular hypertrophy should be trained differently than someone looking to improve muscular power. Also, a program for a beginner will be less intense than that for someone who has been working out for several years. Now that we have reviewed the major stages of an exercise program, let's return to the initial conditioning stage and review basic guidelines that should be followed when working with beginners.

Working Out: The First 8-12 weeks

One of the first things we notice when a baby learns to walk is that they fall down a lot. Many people assume babies fall down because their muscles aren't yet strong enough. While this correct, there's another reason why this happens.

Going from crawling to walking — whether we're talking literally (as in the case of the baby) or figuratively, such as when you begin something like an exercise program, requires not only that your muscles grow stronger but that other changes take place. These other alterations take place in the brain and nervous system and are referred to as "*neurological* changes." When you first begin to do something new, whether it's jogging, lifting weights, bowling, golfing, etc., your nervous system is inexperienced at the task and doesn't yet know how to coordinate your muscles in the way that produces the best, most efficient movement pattern. It's as if your brain and muscles speak different languages. To help them communicate, changes have to be made within the brain and nervous system such that the muscles can be made to understand what is being *said* to them.

In the gym, it's easy to see who hasn't yet acquired these neurological changes. Look at the people who are doing a bench press with a barbell. If, as they lift the weight, they wobble the barbell back and forth and it looks like one arm is lifting the weight faster then the other arm, that's a usually dead give away. With respect to children, most gains in strength before puberty are in fact due to neurological changes. So how long should it take for these neurological changes to take place? Generally 8-12 weeks, but this can vary depending on the age of the person and how difficult the task one is trying to learn.

Programs for Beginners

It's safe to say that many people hire fitness trainers because they are not sure how to safely improve their fitness and health. They want guidance. They also want *results* and more often than not, they want those results *fast*. This usually creates a dilemma for the fitness trainer because achieving "fast results" – especially with beginners – usually goes hand in hand with increased injury, which, in turn, limits the client's ability to train and reduces the ability of the trainer to earn a living as well as help the client achieve the results they seek. Fitness professionals should be just that – professionals. When faced with a person who has never worked out or has done so infrequently, yet wants a magazine-cover body in a few weeks or months, the trainer should be honest and make the person understand this is unlikely. They should then progress the client slowly so as not to increase injury risk. Programs for beginners need not be strenuous or overly lengthy to be effective. In fact, it's possible to work the entire body effectively in as little as 20-30 minutes.

When designing an exercise program for a beginner, remember that while the muscles may quickly get stronger, the tendons, ligaments and other connective tissues will take longer. This is why trying to achieve quick results often results in injury. Because of this, novices are best suited with single set programs of low resistances and relatively high reps for the first few months.[107] Remember that for the first several weeks, much of the improvements they see are due to *neurological factors*. In other words, it's not so much that the muscles are getting stronger (they do, but not as much as you think) but rather that the brain and nervous system are communicating better with the muscles. A better mind-body connection allows for better coordination of muscle recruitment and efficiency in lifting. Let's now discuss this in terms of weight, sets and reps.

How much weight and how many reps? Novices are best suited with relatively light resistances. This is because injury risk increases as the resistance lifted is increased. However, one does not want to lift a weight so many times that injury results. There is no perfect resistance to use with beginners because everybody will have different abilities. Thus, it's best to choose a weight that can be lifted safely and comfortably for 12-20 times. Some fitness trainers may also choose to make this a "12-20 RM" where RM stands for *repetition maximum*. Repetition maximum is the most weight that a person can lift safely for a certain number of times with good lifting technique. For example, a weight that's equal to 12 RM can only be lifted 12 times with good lifting technique. Determining RM usually means performing multiple sets to obtain the load one is seeking. For the untrained person, this will probably lead to DOMS, which the beginner will not appreciate. Thus, for novices, determining RM may not always be necessary. Another alternative is to determine the load by using the RPE scale. Suppose the person is to perform 12 reps. Choose a weight that you feel is appropriate and ask the person how heavy it feels on a scale from zero-10, where 10 is a super heavy weight and "zero" is very, very easy. Ask them how heavy it feels when they first lift the weight, half way through the set and again at the end of the set. This will give you an idea of how they feel during the entire set. For people with special needs (e.g., arthritis) you may want the intensity to be about 2-3 on the RPE scale, while for a healthy person 5-6 may be appropriate. Everyone is different and as the trainer, your job is to pick an intensity that emphasizes benefits while minimizing risks. While the RPE scale may not be 100% accurate for weight training purposes, with novices, you don't need to be super accurate. Your goal is to get them accustomed to lifting weights, boost their confidence and most importantly, minimize injury.

For beginners, usually 8-12 reps for healthy person's under 50 years of age and 10-15 reps for those older than 50-60 years of age are generally recommend.[1] However, for very low-fit person's, lifting a weight for only 8 reps (8RM) may be too much and increase injury risk. Also, these guidelines are not significantly different than the general guideline of 12-20 repetitions mentioned above. As a rule, the greater the number of reps, the more muscle endurance is improved; while at lower reps, the more strength is gained. For beginners, improvement of strength should not be the primary concern (even though it may be the client's). Instead, the trainer should focus on preparing the client's body for the harder training which will come in the future. For most people this is best accomplished with lighter loads which do not injure the body.

The number of sets to be completed per exercise is often a point of contention among trainers with many believing that several sets (e.g., 3 sets) are superior to single set programs. Many studies do find multiple sets superior for improving strength and hypertrophy; but, does this mean they are *always* best for everyone? Obviously the answer is no. Factors that might necessitate only performing one set may include experience level, time constraints, and health issues (e.g., post heart attack, frail or fibromyalgia). For healthy, sedentary person's, the ACSM recommends one set of 8-12 exercises that target the major muscles of the body.[1] Also, single-set programs have been shown to increase strength in beginners for the first 2 -3 months of training.[107] After a few months, they may have adopted a healthy lifestyle and want to do more. Until that happens, single-set programs may serve the needs of the client best.

Benefits of One Set Programs

Improves strength	Not boring	Easy to work whole body in a single session
Improves muscle endurance	Allows busy people to fit fitness into their life	Safest for those with special needs
Reduces injury risk	Is time efficient	Greater degree of adherence for beginners

For programs requiring multiple sets, the rest periods between them will vary according to the person's goals, age, health concerns as well as their fitness level. A general guideline is for rest periods to range from 30 seconds to 2-5 minutes between sets. This is where the *art* of personal training comes in. As a fitness professional you will rely not only on what the client is telling you about how they feel, but also what you observe during exercise. For example, a person may tell you they feel fine and can do another set; but, you notice their arms shaking during the reps, their breathing erratic and their exercise technique breaking down. All this tells you they may have had enough or need additional rest.

Beginner Strength Program: Basic Guidelines

Resistance	Reps	Sets	Rest between sets	Workouts/wk
Light loads	12-20	1 set for first few months	30 sec to 2 -5 min	2-3

Training Goal: Weight Loss

It's safe to assume that many people will hire personal trainers for weight loss help. In truth, many exercise programs can help people lose weight but to truly achieve this goal, people must cut back slightly on the number of calories they consume. Exercise can help with burning calories; but, exercise does not use as many calories as one might expect. Check the calorie counter on the treadmill next time you work out if you doubt this. You might notice that only 200 or so calories are used after 20 minutes of exercise. That's less than is in many protein bars! Thus, with the exception of huge amounts of activity (that many can't/won't do), exercise alone will probably not lead to long-term weight reduction.

When it comes to weight loss, nutrition (eating fewer calories) is more important than exercise for most people — and is usually the hardest part to do. Much evidence substantiates the fact that if weight loss is to be achieved, one must have consumed fewer calories at the end of the day than that needed by the body. For example, if you consumed 2000 calories today but burned off 2500 calories through exercise, metabolism and other activities, you would have a *calorie deficit* of 500 calories. If you did this for seven days in a row, you would have lost 3500 calories (one pound of fat). Weight loss guidelines usually call for achieving a calorie deficit of between 500-1000 calories a day.[1] While this will likely work, for some, reducing this many calories may be challenging. Others call for a smaller reduction. For example, some research suggests that reducing calories by 300 or 400 calories per day may be optimal for women and men respectively who are trying to lose fat without sacrificing their metabolic rate.[113] Regardless, whatever one chooses, it's important to first determine an approximate number of calories currently consumed and reduce this by a little. Over time, any small reduction in calories will cause the body to use its stored fat and glycogen reserves, resulting in weight loss. Some experts call for losing 10% of initial body weight as a good starting point for weight loss.[1] For example, a client weighing 300 lbs should first attempt to lose 30 lbs. One might tackle this by breaking up 30 lbs into 5 or 10 lb increments. Reduce weight slowly, aiming for 0.5-2 pounds per week. This will help preserve muscle mass and maintain metabolic rate. Some research suggests that losing more than ½ pound per week may slow metabolic rate.[157]

Some people may opt for a special diet program to achieve weight loss. Regardless of one's thoughts on the matter, most diets will probably cause short-term weight loss. This is especially true for those that restrict carbohydrate intake as this promotes glycogen breakdown, releasing water that is stored in the body. Remember, each gram of glycogen used releases about 3 grams of water. In other words, burning off one pound of glycogen releases 3 pounds of water! This is why one of the first signs of weight loss on low carb diets is frequent urination. Interestingly, long term weight loss from carb restriction does not appear to be any better than simply reducing calories.[114] When used long term (>6 months), it appears that people on low carb diets simply eat fewer calories out of boredom with the diet's food choices. One big problem with most diets is that there comes a time when one goes off the diet and returns to old eating habits. This usually results in a regaining of weight. Remind clients that there is a difference between a diet and a life-long change in eating patterns.

Dieting alone is not enough for healthy weight loss. By itself, dieting can lead to significant loss of muscle tissue, which is unhealthy. With respect to exercise, both aerobic and anaerobic activities should be included. It usually won't matter what you do first – strength or cardio. Just remember to warm the client up first. As a rule, activities should incorporate large muscle groups (chest, back and legs) to maximize calorie usage. Depending on their needs/limitations, ADL-type activities may also be included to improve quality of life. Since boredom as well as lack of strength and endurance may be issues to consider, *circuit training* may be most appropriate for these individuals when starting an exercise program. Usually 8-10 different exercises that target the major muscles of the body should be included in the circuit. Adding in a bike or treadmill to the circuit will increase calorie use and enhance the aerobic aspect of the circuit. For those with joint issues, pool exercise may be appropriate. Keeping exercise intensity low will ensure that the deconditioned person can sustain at least 30 minutes of physical activity. When designing an exercise circuit, keep in mind that very large people may not easily fit in some strength machines.

Body Fat Testing: Yes or No?

The notion of performing body composition testing on people looking for weight loss is controversial in some circles. Some say do it as it will help spur the client to future results when he/she sees what he/she has accomplished. Others say not to do it as it may embarrass the client. Also, in the case of body fat calipers, some clients may not like being pinched by people they barely know – especially those of the opposite gender. In addition, it may be difficult to perform some tests (e.g., calipers) in those who are very overweight. Personally, I explain the benefits of body composition testing and let the client make the call. If the person says no, that's fine. They may change their mind at some point after thinking it over. The big issue is that we never want to make another person feel uncomfortable. Presenting yourself in the most professional manner you can will go a long way in making others feel at ease around you, which in the long run, will help you help your clients to greater success.

Training Goal: Muscular Endurance

Muscle endurance is defined as the ability of a muscle to exert force for extended periods of time and comes into play during a host of activities ranging from carrying groceries to running triathlons. Strength training can improve muscular endurance and aerobic exercise performance. To improve muscular endurance it is necessary to use lighter resistances, usually 12-15 RM and perform 1 to 3 sets per exercise.[78] Thus, the intensity of exercise is generally low when training for muscle endurance. In addition, the rest periods should also be short, generally less than 30 seconds between sets.[78] Short rest periods are needed because it most simulates endurance activities like a marathon. Training for this effect mainly taxes the aerobic (oxidative) energy system and type I muscle fibers.

Training Goal: Muscle Hypertrophy

When training for muscle size, the volume (weight x reps x sets) of exercise tends be greater than that for muscle endurance. In general, the resistance used should be between 8RM-12RM. Because heavier resistances are used, the rest periods between sets tend to be longer, with 30 seconds to 1.0-1.5 minutes being common.[78] One key issue though is to stress the muscle again before it has fully recovered.[181] As the person becomes more fit, less rest time may be required between sets. Also as the person improves, performing one set may not be enough to foster the results he/she seeks. Studies show that hypertrophy training tends to elicit greater release in GH and testosterone compared to those designed to improve muscle strength only.[181] In addition, multiple exercises per body part appear to be better than single sets at producing hypertrophy.[76,77] During hypertrophy, much metabolic stress is placed on the anaerobic energy system (the aerobic system is used also). These programs usually target both type I and type II fibers. While not normally discussed, it is possible for type I fibers to undergo some hypertrophy. However, the degree to which these fibers grow is less than that of type II fibers.[77] Interestingly, the biochemical process by which hypertrophy occurs appears to be different between fiber types. Specifically, type II fibers undergo hypertrophy mostly because of an increase in protein synthesis. Type I fibers, on the other hand, grow because of a reduction in protein breakdown.[111] In addition, there is evidence that traditionally-used bodybuilding programs (higher volume, lighter weights) tend to hypertrophy both type I and type II fibers. This is contrasted by that of powerlifting which seems to result in less type I fiber hypertrophy.[77] Hypertrophy-based programs almost certainly also facilitate the conversion of type IIb fibers to the more athletic type IIa fibers as well.

How Long Before Hypertrophy Occurs?

People will often ask you how long before their muscles start to grow. In reality the body responds to strength training after just a few workouts.[108] However, changes in muscle fiber cross sectional area and hypertrophy usually require at least 8 weeks of consistent training.[77] Thus, it may take as long as 8 weeks before people see any noticeable changes in physique.

Training Goal: Muscle Power/ Muscle Strength

Muscle strength and muscle power are not the same thing. Strength is the exertion of force over time. Power, on the other hand, is basically explosive strength. In other words, it packs a big punch but doesn't last long (e.g., 30 seconds). Nevertheless, the protocols to improve both power and strength are very similar. In general, improving strength or power requires very heavy weights (~1-8 RM), and comparatively long rest periods (2-5 minutes) between sets.[78] In its purest sense, power-oriented workouts recruit mostly the ATP/CP system. As a result, muscles trained for strength and power tend to be different in terms of their biochemical adaptations. For example, endurance-trained muscles tend to have more numerous (and bigger) mitochondria and greater capillary densities than that of strength/power trained muscles.

Quick Reference: Determining Strength Training Experience[112]

Experience Level	Are they working out?	Length of training	Days per week to lift	Intensity of program
Beginner	No or just started	<2 months	< 1-2 days/wk	Very little
Moderate experience	Yes	2-6 months	<2-3 days/wk	Moderate
Experienced	Yes	> 1 year	>3-4 days/wk	High

Weight Lifting Belts

It's almost a rite of passage when a person gets their first weight set that they also purchase a weightlifting belt. But, are they needed? In theory, weightlifting belts help by increasing the pressure inside the abdominal cavity (intraabominal pressure) which helps stabilize the lower core musculature and spinal cord which in theory reduces low back injuries. Some lifter's also feel belts increase lifting performance.[128] Studies of weightlifting belt usage, however, have noted that many gym members use belts for the wrong reasons.[128] The National Strength and Conditioning Association (NSCA) recommends that weightlifting belts only be used for maximal or near maximal lifts that stress the low back.[78] Trainers should also remember that studies of weightlifting belts have not consistently found that they improve performance or reduce injury risk.[128] One possible negative side effect of using such belts on a regular basis is that they may *weaken* the back muscles as the body grows accustomed to the added help that belts might provide. People who experience pain during lifts should not rely on a belt. Pain is a signal that something is wrong. In this case, the pain-eliciting exercise should be halted and the lifter referred to his/her physician who can make the appropriate diagnosis.

Periodization

All fitness trainers should have at least a working knowledge of periodization and how it can help improve people's fitness levels. In reality, while never mentioning it, periodization is what we have been reviewing in this chapter up to this point. Periodization refers to breaking up workouts into different periods or cycles. During each cycle, the weight, reps, sets, exercise selection, rest periods and exercise order chosen are specific to help reduce injury and improve fitness levels. During some of these periods, the exercise stress is low while at others, the stress is higher. At the start of the program, the stress is kept low (e.g., one set) and not specific to any body part or goal; as one progresses and gets stronger, the stress of the workout is increased and becomes more focused.

Central to periodization is how the body adapts to the stress applied to it. The body adapts to any stress in stages. The process that describes these stages is referred to as the *General Adaptation Syndrome* (GAS) first proposed by the scientist, Hans Selye. According to GAS, the body goes through three phases as it adapts. The *alarm phase* is the first stage. It is here that the person tends to experience DOMS and muscle stiffness as the body tries to cope with the stress of the new exercise program. Exercise performance may fluctuate for several weeks during this stage as the body adapts.

During the *resistance phase*, the body slowly begins to adapt to the exercise and begins to grow stronger due to both muscle growth enhancements and biochemical changes as well as to various neurological alterations. If, however, the same stimulus is applied too long or is increased too fast, the body will begin to break down and become weaker and more prone to injury. This is called the *exhaustion phase*. It is during the exhaustion phase that overtraining syndrome might become evident. The trick for trainers is to keep people in the adaptation phase and avoid the exhaustion phase at all cost. The best way to do this is by altering programs periodically, using periodization.

Generally, there are three major cycles in periodization. A *macrocycle* is the largest cycle and encompasses a whole year of training. Each macrocycle is made up of several *mesocycles* which can last from many weeks to several months. Each mesocycle, is, in turn, made up of many *microcycles* which are about a week long. Obviously, periodization takes planning. Remember, a person's fitness level, physical limitations, age and time commitment will all dictate how long these cycles really last. For example, you could have microcycles lasting a month.

Within the cycles of periodization are also several distinct parts called *periods* and *phases*. Let's review the periods and phases now, keeping in mind that while periodization was originally designed for "athletes," its principles can be applied to anyone. Athlete or not, the major goals of periodization are reduction in injury and boredom and optimal physical performance over time.

The *preparatory period* is usually taken to be the first stage of periodization and is where many people will focus most of their efforts. It is here that the preparation work is done to ready the person for his/her ultimate goal or competition. This period is composed of three distinct phases: hypertrophy phase, strength phase and power phase.

In the *hypertrophy phase*, to goal is to provide a foundation of muscular hypertrophy and endurance. Notice that endurance is part of this phase. Untrained muscles usually have little endurance. During this phase the sets can be anywhere from 1-6 depending on fitness level. The loads are generally light/moderate (8-12 RM) and the reps somewhat higher (12-20). Depending on fitness level, age and health issues, the sets, reps and resistances used may be less than this. For those new to exercise, it is not always necessary to determine an exact RM range. Doing so may expose people to injury or increase DOMS. The important thing for beginners is to not overwhelm them but still challenge them enough to fatigue the muscles within 12-20 reps. The intensity during this phase is generally low while volume of exercise (weight x reps x sets) is high. While workouts usually occur 2-3 times a week, use your good judgment when deciding this. This phase may last up to 6 weeks and can even go longer than this if you deem it necessary.

During the *strength phase*, the intensity of the workout is increased. Generally 3-5 sets of 4-10 reps, at 6-12RM, 2-4 days a week are used. For many people, periodization can stop here (or at the hypertrophy phase). Once a person reaches their desired strength, endurance or hypertrophy, it is not always necessary to progress to the power phase.

Power is the application of strength explosively. How many people can sprint full speed, non-stop for 20 minutes? Nobody! As such, power does not last very long and usually exhausts itself in 30 seconds or less. Nevertheless, power is indispensable to the successful completion of many sports. During the power phase of the preparatory period, the intensity of the workouts increase and become more specific to what the person's athletic goals are. Also, the volume of the workouts decreases accordingly. This is so as not to injure or overwhelm the athlete as his/her competition approaches.

Usually the power phase requires performing 2-3 sets of 2-5 reps at an intensity of 75-95% of 1RM.[78] While some ADLs may require muscle power (i.e., crossing a busy street), for non-athletes, the trainer needs to use his/her good judgment on whether to include this phase. When working with non-athletes, examine the person's goals, ADLs, injuries, age and other limitations before attempting the power phase.

Following the power phase, some trainers may include a brief active rest period (*first transition period*) to give the person a break from the rigors of tough training. This may last for a week or two. After this, is the *competition period*. With respect to athletes, the competition period is the time they are actively participating in their sport. The focus here is not necessarily on exhaustive workouts but rather on more sports-oriented items that are specific to their successful sports performance. During this time, the intensity of exercise is high (e.g., 85% - >90% 1RM) while volume is low with usually 1-3 sets of 1-8 reps performed. This period may last for the season of their sport. As such, it will be necessary to manipulate frequency, intensity and volume to accommodate their sport and not overtax the person. The goal here is to keep them at peak performance for as long as possible. For non-athletes the competition phase is usually not needed.

Following the competition period is a time of active rest called the *second transition period* in which the person takes a break from intense training and participates in recreational activities generally between 1-4 weeks.[78] After this, goals can be reassessed and another macrocycle can be planned for the following year.

Is this all there is to periodization? Absolutely not! Periodization is a complex topic and there are many good books available to help those who want to learn more. The goal here was to provide a foundation from which to build upon. It is important to remember that periodization is really a fluid concept rather than one that is fixed and unyielding. As such, the rules given here for sets, reps and weight are generally textbook guidelines and should not be taken as gospel for all people. Fitness trainers are more likely to encounter untrained novices than athletes. Age, desire to train, health issues, goals and fear to name a few will all impact how quickly one progresses. While most of your clients may not progress as fast as was outlined here, periodization can help all people achieve greater results over time. If your first rules of thumb are *do no harm* and *progress people slowly*, periodization can be a great benefit to your clients and separate you from others who do not use this powerful training tool.

Periodization Quick Reference

Period/Phase	Details/goals
Preparatory Period	Builds foundation for future training
Hypertrophy Phase	Muscular hypertrophy and muscular endurance. High volume, low resistances
Strength Phase	Increase strength. Intensity increases/volume decreases
Power Phase*	Develop explosive strength. Intensity increases/volume decreases
Competition Period*	High intensity/low volume. Sports specific movements
Active Rest (transition) Period	Recreational activities. Gives body time to recuperate

* May not be needed in non-athletes

Types of Strength Programs

There are many different types of strength training programs. This section will review some of the more common protocols used by people. Keep in mind that variations of each program exist and research does not generally find one system better than another for all people. All programs have their place and their limitations. The key for the exercise professional is to decide which program balances safety, effectiveness and appropriateness for the person he/she is working with.

Single Set Programs: Single set programs are typically total body programs and some of the easiest to design. They usually consist of performing only one set of an exercise per body part. For example, one might do a chest press, followed by a lat pull down, followed by a leg press, etc. After completing one exercise for each of the major muscle groups, the person is finished. The resistance used is generally heavy enough to fatigue the muscle within about 12-15 reps (i.e., 12-15RM). Single-set programs share some things in common with circuit training but generally do not incorporate a cardio component. Cardio can be performed separately, either after the single-set program or on an alternate day depending on time, goals, fatigue level and health profile. Single set programs are usually safest for beginners.

Circuit Training: This mode of strength training is a total body program that entails that the lifter use lighter resistances (e.g., 12-20 RM or 40% to 60% 1 RM) and move from one exercise to another with little or no rest in between. If rest periods are used, they are kept short, lasting no more than 30 seconds. Generally 9-15 exercises targeting the major muscle groups make up a circuit; however this can vary considerably. A well designed circuit ensures that no single muscle group receives any undue stress. If one completes the circuit and has the time and energy for more, the circuit can be performed again. While machines are typically used in circuits, this rule is not fixed. It's possible to have free weight circuits or circuits that use both machines and free weights. Stability balls, elastic tubing, medicine balls, etc. can also be used. The design of an exercise circuit is limited only by one's imagination. While typically considered to improve only strength, aerobic capacity (VO2max) also improves with circuit training. Some research suggests that circuit training can improve aerobic capacity by 4% - 8% in men and women respectively over the course of 20 weeks of training.[142] Other research, though, notes that aerobic capacity may improve even more up to 51%.[143] For added benefit and variety, treadmills, bikes, etc. can also be added to the exercise circuit. Besides being fun and not boring, circuit training offers a reduced chance of injury relative to other strength training protocols. This makes it a very attractive option for beginners. Another major benefit is that circuits are deemed by the ACSM as the safest type of workout regimen for those with a number of medical issues ranging from heart disease, hypertension, cancer, bleeding disorders (e.g., hemophilia), and arthritis, to name a few.[141] Circuit training also lends itself well to those with limited time to exercise and can even be quite challenging if needed (e.g., "boot camp" type workouts).

Isometric Programs: Isometric programs involve pressing or pulling against immovable objects. For example, pressing the hands together on front of the chest is an isometric chest exercise. Another name for this is *static contractions*. Isometrics may be employed in some physical therapy settings to help deconditioned/injured individuals. But, they are almost certainly progressed to more challenging workouts eventually. While isometrics may be performed alongside more traditional movements (concentric + eccentric), they are usually not the primary focus of an exercise program. Isometric exercise can improve strength; however the strength appears to be limited to the joint angle used during the movement. Some research also hints that longer recovery periods between sets may be required when performing isometric movements.[181] Also, isometrics may increase blood pressure more than traditional strength training programs. This might make isometrics inappropriate for those with heart disease and/or high blood pressure.

Multiple Set Programs: Multiple set programs entail performing more than one set of an exercise. For example, a person might do 3 sets of 10 reps of a bench press, lat pull down, leg press, etc. Rest periods lasting anywhere from less than 30 seconds to up to 5 minutes are typically used between sets, depending on the training goal (i.e., less rest for muscular endurance; more rest for strength and power). Within the multiple set arena, variations are possible such as keeping the load constant or increasing/decreasing the load on subsequent sets.

Fitness professionals continually debate which is best to do – single sets or multiple sets – for improving strength. Both systems will of course work but the question should be expanded to include the person one is dealing with. For the beginner, research suggests that multiple sets can produce greater strength than single sets.[144] However other research suggests that single set programs work just as well.[142] Regardless of which produces greater strength, the issue should be placed within the greater context that untrained people may not enjoy exercise. Forcing these people to perform multiple sets may result in a greater drop-out rate. Also, beginners, who believe the efficacy of multiple sets may put themselves at greater risk of injury because of improper technique or lack of knowledge of the proper application of training variables. Also, while multiple sets may develop more strength than single sets in beginners, the difference is often not a lot.[144] Because of this and the increased time commitment coupled with possible increase in injury, single-set programs may be best/safest for the first couple of months of training. Beyond this though, multiple sets are superior.

Split Routine Programs: Split routines are a catch-all phrase for any program that splits training into separate days. Each day, a different body part or parts is focused on. The advantage of a split routine is that one can focus more on individual body parts. For example, one might spend one day working just chest and biceps. Because they allow for greater intensity yet don't require a person to spend hours in the gym, they are quite popular with bodybuilders and athletes. Split routines also allow more rest between workouts. Many of the other programs described in this section are variations of split routines. The downside is that split routines typically mean we spend more days in the gym, which may not be the best for beginners. Technically, one could work out 7 days in a row if he/she really wanted to. While popular among advanced lifter's, what little research there is hints that this may not be the best way for novices to train. For example, one study looked at 5 months of training with either a whole body program or a split routine in 30 untrained young women.[146] In spite of the differences in routines, similar results were obtained.

Super Set Programs: When someone does a superset, they may be performing one of two separate, but similar types of programs. One type of supersetting involves performing two exercises back to back that target opposing muscle groups. For example, one might perform a leg extension followed by a leg curl. Typically, little or no rest is taken between the exercises. By targeting opposing muscle groups, one muscle rests while the other is working.

Another type of supersetting involves performing 2 or 3 different exercises for the same muscle group with little rest. For example, one might do a set of dumbbell biceps curls, followed by a set of spider curls. Supersetting is popular with bodybuilders and those who have limited time to work out.

Push/Pull Programs: In a push/pull program, the lifter generally performs all of the pushing exercises (bench press, leg press, etc.) on one day followed by all the pulling movements (lat pull down, biceps curl, etc.) on another day. Thus, push/pull programs can be considered a type of *split routine*. A variation of this program is to perform a pushing movement followed immediately by a pulling exercise. In this respect, push/pull programs are very similar to supersetting. One advantage of push/pull programs is that they are time efficient, allowing multiple sets to be performed with little time.

Pyramiding Programs: With pyramid-type programs, the lifter usually begins with a light resistance that he/she can lift for about 10-12 reps (10RM -12 RM). On subsequent sets, the lifter increases the weight (by 2.5-10 lbs), which results in a decrease in the number of reps that can be performed. Ultimately, the lifter reaches the top of the pyramid and can only perform one rep. After this, the weight is reduced (by 2.5-10 lbs), resulting in more reps being able to be performed. At the bottom of the pyramid, the lifter is once again, back to his/her starting point. One variation of this program entails that the lifter perform only half the pyramid. From this, we get the frequently used terms "up pyramiding" (i.e., ascending pyramid program) and "down pyramiding" (i.e., descending pyramid program). An up pyramid is when you start with a light resistance (e.g., 12 RM) and gradually increase the resistance. A down pyramid is the opposite – starting with a heavy resistance (e.g., 10RM) and gradually reducing the weight on subsequent lifts. Another name for down pyramiding is "stripping" because we strip off the weight during each set. Everyone has ideas on which is better, but, little research proves conclusively the superiority of one system over another. Both have their place in a strength training program and periodically alternating between systems may produce better results than either program alone. For beginners, though, performing either system is likely to be difficult, resulting in DOMS and, in theory, may ramp up injuries.

Eccentric Only Training Programs: This type of program consists of only performing eccentric muscle actions ("negatives"). While greater force production does appear to occur during eccentric muscle actions, interestingly, studies that directly compare concentric only muscle actions to eccentric only muscle actions and their ability to increase overall strength are mixed with some finding that eccentrics are better and others which find no difference.[77,147] Other research suggests that eccentric only reps may be superior in the development of muscle hypertrophy.[148] Still other research finds that performing a heavy eccentric rep just prior to performing a concentric rep enhances the lifter's 1RM.[151] The reasons for this effect are unknown but may be at least partially due to greater neurological stimulation caused by eccentric reps.[151] For those who wish to try this mode of training, there are several options. Some computerized strength machines allow the lifter to enter a light resistance during the concentric phase and a very heavy resistance during the eccentric phase. It's also possible to perform only-eccentric reps by using a lifting partner or, if using a machine, by lifting the heavy weight with both limbs and lowering it with only one limb (e.g., leg extension). Lifting partners might also apply additional manual resistance during the eccentric phase. Regardless of how you look at it, performing only eccentric reps is an advanced form of strength training and may result in injury (e.g., muscle tearing away from the bone) if used in beginners. In my opinion, this type of training should not be performed unless the lifter has been consistently involved in heavy strength training for at least a year.

Super Slow Type Programs: In super slow programs, the weight is lifted very slowly. One popular method calls for 10 seconds to be spent lifting the weight and 5 seconds lowering the weight.[149] Some research does suggests that super slow training may augment strength in untrained individuals.[150] Other research suggests that super slow may not be optimal when used for weight loss in experienced lifter's because fewer calories may be used.[149] Conversely, by forcing the individual to perform the exercise slowly, in theory, super slow programs may lead to fewer injuries.

Rhabdomyolysis

Rhabdomyolysis (rhab-doe-my-ol-la-sis) is a serious condition whereby muscle cells rupture from an overwhelming stress that's applied too fast for the body to adapt. When exercise is the stress, it is called *exertional* or *exercise-induced* rhabdomyolysis. After skeletal muscles rupture, they release their cellular contents into the blood which can result in sometimes fatal outcomes. It is possible to die from rhabdomyolysis.[184] Exercise in hot environments as well as activities that focus on eccentric muscle actions also appear to increase its incidence. It's also important to note that even a single session of extreme activity can cause this condition.[153] It's difficult to determine what intensity level of exercise is needed to induce rhabdomyolysis. In one case report the syndrome occurred in a 29-year-old man who reported performing 30 sit-ups a day for 5 days.[155] This leaves open the possibility that some people may be more susceptible to rhabdomyolysis than others. Indeed, some medical conditions (e.g., sickle cell anemia) do appear to increase risk.[154] Cases of exertional rhabdomyolysis have been reported in the military, as well as in firemen, law enforcement trainees, football players, bodybuilders and marathoners.[152,182] In addition, case reports also have documented rhabdomyolysis arising as a direct result from overzealous personal trainers who push their clients too hard.[153] While medical tests can diagnosis this condition quite rapidly, fitness professionals may overlook it or mistake it for DOMS or overuse injuries. One classic sign that may help its recognition is the presence of dark-colored (think coke-a-cola) urine.[152] This is a sign of blood in the urine. Other signs that highlight the seriousness of this condition can include kidney failure, heart attack and intense muscle pain, muscle weakness and swelling. Muscle soreness is typically said to occur sooner (12-24 hrs) than DOMS-related muscle soreness. (24-72 hrs).[152] This pain usually results in a loss of movement through a muscle's normal ROM. Why the condition occurs is not well understood but may be related to instances when energy needs exceed the body's ability to make ATP. [154] Not everyone who has dark-colored urine or has experienced rhabdomyolysis dies. Also, while we have only discussed exercise-induced rhabdomyolysis, know that it can occur following other types of trauma such as car accidents. Some cholesterol-lowering medications may also cause this condition. Because most people have never heard of rhabdomyolysis, its recognition is something all fitness professionals should be aware of and educate people about.

Interval Training Programs: These programs alternate between intense and less intense efforts. For example, following a proper warm up, one might run on a treadmill for 30 seconds at a fast pace, followed by walking for 3 minutes at a slower pace. In theory, programs such as these may cut down on overuse injuries by reducing the overall time muscles are subjected to high degrees of stress. Interval training programs can also improve aerobic fitness levels. In addition, these programs might also result in more calories being used in a workout. For example, just as your car is less efficient (uses more energy) when you drive in stop-and-go city traffic, we use more energy when we alternate between intense and less intense exercise levels. If designing an interval training program, it's generally wise to make the rest period 2 to 3 times longer than the work period. For example, if the person runs on a treadmill for 1 minute at a fast pace, that person should walk for 2 to 3 minutes at a slower pace. Regardless of the benefits, because of the stressful nature that many of these programs require, they are usually are not appropriate for beginners or those with health issues (e.g. heart disease, arthritis). In beginners and those with health issues, interval training might increase injuries.

Chapter 9

EXERCISE TECHNIQUE

This chapter will deal with the proper way to perform a variety of strength training exercises. Each exercise is broken down according to the major muscles used, spotting tips and various comments and suggestions regarding the exercise in question. To facilitate learning, various movements are also broken down into their concentric and eccentric phases. While there are hundreds of different types of strength training activities, this chapter will deal with many of the more common (and some not so common) movements that fitness trainers should be familiar with.

SEATED MACHINE CHEST PRESS

Primary Muscles Worked: Pectoralis major, anterior deltoids, triceps.

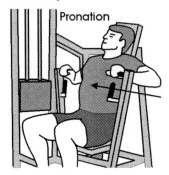

> **Quick Tip:** The neutral grip is usually easier on the shoulders than the pronated grip shown here.

Exercise Technique: Adjust the seat height to where the handles are about parallel with the nipple line of chest. Usually the feet are on the floor or floor plate of the machine, with the thighs parallel to floor. Grasp the handgrips keeping the forearms parallel to the floor. Wrists should not be bent. Wrap the thumbs around handgrips. The starting point is when elbows are in line with shoulders. The elbows should not be behind the torso. If lifting heavy weights, pull the shoulder blades together (retract scapula) and try to maintain this retraction for the duration of the exercise. With lighter weights, pulling the shoulder blades together may not be needed. Concentric phase: Slowly press forward and stop just before the elbows lock out (i.e., a "soft lockout"). Hold for a second. Eccentric phase: Slowly lower weight to the starting position; however, do not let elbows travel past the point of the torso (or midline of the body).

Spotting: Wrists should be firm/straight and not bent. Thumbs should be wrapped around the handgrips. The fitness professional can stand in front of the machine making sure the lifter's form is correct, or stand either behind or on the side of the machine. Standing behind or on the side may be easier to cue the person where to halt the eccentric phase of the exercise.

Comments & Suggestions: The machine chest press is a multi-joint exercise designed to mimic the bench press with free weights. Many chest press machines have two handgrip positions. The picture depicted here shows the more traditional, pronated position with the palms facing down. People with shoulder injuries may find the neutral position (with palms facing each other) easier on the shoulders. Some machines have a pedal or bar close to the floor upon which the feet can press against, which brings the handles to a safe position for starting the exercise. This negates having to reach back, bringing the elbows past the torso, which can exacerbate shoulder injuries. On some versions of this machine, it is possible to maintain contact between the feet and the bar/pedal. Doing so may stop the handles from traveling back too far, saving the shoulder from potential harm. This can also teach beginners the correct ROM of the exercise. The normal convention is to exhale when lifting the weight and inhale during the lowering phase. Novices may have trouble coordinating breathing and lifting. If this happens, instruct the person to count or talk during the lift. The end result is the same – maintaining proper blood pressure and avoiding the Valsalva maneuver.

BARBELL BENCH PRESS

Primary Muscles Worked: Pectoralis major and minor, anterior deltoids, triceps, serratus anterior.

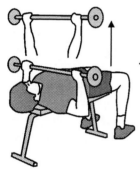

Quick Tip: Retract the shoulder blades prior to performing this exercise with heavy resistances.

Exercise Technique: The barbell should have equal weight on both sides and be secured by collars. Adjust the height of the barbell such that there is a slight bend in the elbows when you grasp the barbell in the supine position. When supine on the bench, the barbell should be lined up with the eyes. The rest of the body should be evenly distributed on the bench with feet on floor at least shoulder width apart, if not a little wider. Feet can be under the knees or a little in front of them. The spine should be neutral and not hyper-extended. Grasp barbell with a pronated grip, wrapping the thumbs around the bar. The wrists are straight and not bent. The grip should be about shoulder-width apart or a little wider. Hands and elbows are in line with each other. Begin by lifting the barbell off of its suspension hooks to a position in line with the chest. Arms are straight but elbows are not fully locked. Eccentric phase: Lower the bar slowly, stopping when the elbow is at the level of the shoulder. At the end of the eccentric phase the forearms should be perpendicular to the ground (i.e., 90° bend in arms). Do not bounce the barbell off of the chest. Pause for a second. Concentric phase: Slowly press the barbell upward and stop just before the elbows are locked out. Repeat for the desired number of repetitions.

Spotting: It is common for the trainer to stand behind the head of the lifter during this exercise. The trainer who spots for this exercise usually will be in the athletic position (abs tight, knees slightly bent). Trainers usually ask if the lifter needs a "lift off" or help getting the barbell off the hooks to its proper location over the chest. If the lifter answers yes, spotters often use an *alternated grip* (one hand is supinated; the other pronated). The same grip is used at the end of the set if helping re-rack the barbell. Spotting is more than just helping with the lift off. It also involves spotting errors in lifting technique, giving verbal feedback and encouragement and watching for signs that the lifter may be in danger (e.g., wobbling or unstable, shaking arms, arching back, holding breath). At some point during the concentric phase the lifter may reach the *sticking point* (the most difficult point of the exercise). The lifter may need help from his/her spotter during this time. Spotters should also always ask the lifter how many reps he/she can perform so they have an idea when the lifter may need help. Remove weight plates from the barbell evenly. Taking too much weight off only one side of the barbell may cause the barbell to flip over and cause injury.

Comments & Suggestions: The technique described above is commonly performed by many people; but, in some cases, this may result in rotator cuff shoulder injury. Thus, a more narrow grip is sometimes advocated.[136] An added bonus to a narrow grip is that it also tends to place more emphasis on the pecs than does a wider grip. Some call for lowering the barbell until it touches the chest. For most people this is not needed as it might cause or exacerbate shoulder injuries. One way to teach how far to descend is to place a rolled up towel on the lifter's chest. When used, the elbows are usually in line with the shoulder when the bar contacts with the towel. Those involved in Olympic and Powerlifter's, though, train differently and need to adhere to the rules of their sports. When calculating weight lifted, remember to count the Olympic bar (45 lbs) and the collars. One difference between barbells and dumbbells is that because the barbell is a single weight, it is easier to balance than dumbbells. As such, people generally can lift more weight with barbells. Thus, it may be prudent to start with barbells and progress to dumbbells. Also, the argument can be made that dumbbells allow for a greater range of motion which might lead to greater overall muscular strength. The head of the lifter should be kept on the bench at all time. Some research suggests that lifting the head off the bench decreases the weight that can be lifted.[137] Strength trainers who lift heavy weights should be aware of a condition called "effort thrombosis" in which blood clots form from repeated trauma of the axillosubclavian vein in the upper body.[172] While rare, this condition may be more frequent in bodybuilders and heavy strength trainers. Signs can include pain and swelling in neck and shoulder, coupled with limited mobility. This condition requires immediate medical attention.

Common Bench Press Mistakes

Error	Reason
Bouncing barbell off chest	Barbell might crack sternum or cause other injury. It also means lifter did not take advantage of strength-enhancing eccentric phase of the exercise.
Lifting too much weight	Golgi tendon organ (GTO) relaxes muscles if it detects an injury will result from lifting too much weight
Lifting too fast	Places excessive stress on joints, increasing injury risk
Arching the low back	Places excessive stress on low back muscles and spinal cord
Not wrapping thumbs around bar	Barbell might roll out of hands
Bending wrists	Places excessive forces on delicate wrist bones
Raising head off of bench	Stresses cervical neck area. May cause neck injury
Shoulders arching to earlobes (seated chest press only)	Incorrect technique. May signify shoulders performing more work than they should.
Holding breath	Valsalva Maneuver. Might increases BP to dangerous levels
Grip too wide	The wider the grip the more stress on the shoulders
Locking out elbows	May increase injury to elbow joint

DUMBBELL BENCH PRESS

Primary Muscles Worked: Pectoralis major and minor, anterior deltoids, triceps, serratus anterior.

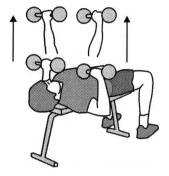

> **Quick Tip:** During the eccentric phase, stop when the elbows are at or just a little below the torso.

Exercise Technique: Grasp two dumbbells of equal weight and sit on a stable exercise bench with dumbbells resting on your thighs. If necessary, perform hip flexion to use the thighs to help lift the dumbbells to shoulder level prior to lying supine on the bench. Lie supine on the bench, with feet on floor at least shoulder width apart, if not wider. Head, shoulders and buttocks should be evenly distributed on the bench. Wrists should be straight, not bent. The dumbbells should be at chest level, aligned with the nipple line. At all times during the exercise, keep the thumbs wrapped around the dumbbells. Rotate arms such that elbows are pointed away from the body (i.e., are lateral to the torso). The elbows should be at the level of the shoulders. The forearms should be perpendicular to floor and elbows in line with shoulders. Concentric phase: Slowly press dumbbells upward. Don't allow the dumbbells to sway back and forth or lose control of them at any point in the ROM. Press until soft lockout is reached. Do not arch the low back or remove the feet from the floor during the lift. Eccentric phase: Slowly lower the dumbbells to the starting point and repeat for the desired number of repetitions. At the end of the exercise at the bottom of the last eccentric phase, rotate the elbows inward toward the body, sit up slowly and rest the dumbbells on the thighs.

Spotting: It is common for trainers to be positioned behind the person's head, low to the ground during this exercise. During the eccentric phase trainers may place their hands at the height of the shoulders to cue the lifter not to lower his/her elbows past this point. During the concentric phase, trainers may grasp the wrists of the client to help him/her steady the dumbbells and reduce injury. Do not pull the dumbbells up by the wrists of the lifter as this may result in shoulder injury especially if the lifter is not expecting it. Ask the lifter how he/she wants to be spotted ahead of time. With very heavy dumbbells it may be necessary to hand the lifter the dumbbells prior to performing the exercise. If this occurs, the spotter should *not* hold the dumbbell by the handgrip. Doing so prevents the lifter from grasping the dumbbell safely. Rather, grasp each end of the dumbbell and hand it to the lifter.

Comments & Suggestions: It's important to maintain a closed grip on dumbbells at all times during the exercise. Failure to do so may lead to injury. Note the height of the bench. A bench that is too high may cause one to arch the lower back. If this happens, place the feet on a raised platform or an aerobic step to alleviate this problem. Placing the feet on the bench is also an option but remember that when the feet are on the bench, the lifter's base of support is narrower which might lead to falling off the bench. The dumbbells do not have to clank together at the top of the lift. Doing so may cause the paint of some dumbbells to flake off which can get in the eyes of lifter's. Depending on shoulder stability and pain-free ROM, the dumbbells can be kept in the same plane of motion or moved closer together during the concentric phase. Lifter's sometimes lower the dumbbells to points where the elbows are far below the torso. They do this because they want to "feel the stretch." But, this practice removes stress from the chest muscles and places more stress on the shoulder joint – one of the weakest areas of the body. This is why one does not have to lower dumbbells past the torso line for this exercise to be effective. This exercise can also be performed with a neutral grip where the elbows are closer to the body and palms facing each other. This grip generally places less stress on the shoulder. Some people may, at the end of the lift, simply drop the weights on the floor while they are supine on the bench. This can lead to shoulder injury and is not advised. In addition, anyone nearby may be injured as well. Technically, dumbbells are more difficult to handle than barbells.

Inner and Outer Pecs: Do They Exist?

Some say that a wider grip on the bench press works more of the "outer pecs" while a narrow grip targets the "inner pecs." However, the inner and outer pecs are really an urban legend. The pecs are made up of the pectoralis major muscle and pectoralis minor. Hand placement though does appear to activate different aspects of the chest and this is probably where the confusion arose from. One study noted that a wider grip activated more of the lower aspect of the pec while a more narrow grip targeted the more of the upper portion of the chest muscle.[127]

PUSH UPS ON THE STABILITY BALL

Primary Muscles Used: Pectoralis major, anterior deltoids, triceps, serratus anterior, posterior deltoids, rectus abdominis, core musculature.

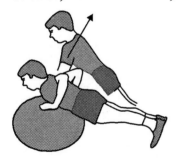

Quick Tip: Be proficient at regular push ups before attempting. Placing the feet closer together increases the difficulty of this exercise.

Exercise Technique: Obtain a properly inflated stability ball and place the hands on the top outer, upper sides of the ball, about shoulder width apart with fingers oriented downward, to the sides of the ball. In this position the elbows will be closer to the body and not flared out at the sides. The legs are extended and at shoulder width apart or wider with bodyweight on toes. Eccentric phase: Slowly lower the upper torso down to the ball while keeping the ball in line with the chest. Halt the movement when the elbows are at the level of the torso or when comfortable. Concentric phase: Press down on the ball, lifting the torso to starting point, while again, keeping the ball in line with the chest. Stop just before the elbows lock out. Hold position for a second or two. Repeat.

Spotting: The low back should not slouch downward. The head should stay neutral, neither lifting up nor turning to the sides. The hands may slide off the ball if sweaty.

Comments & Suggestions: This is an advanced form of push ups that challenges the entire core musculature and requires considerable strength and endurance. This can also be an effective shoulder stabilizing exercise for overall shoulder health. This movement requires considerable core strength. The core is sometimes mentioned in relation to the abs and low back muscles; however, the core really includes all the muscles of the trunk. The gluteals, for example, are part of the core. Another version of this exercise is to perform the push up with hands on the floor and ankles resting on the ball. One limiting factor to performing this movement may be on the forces experienced on the wrists. While it may seem that this exercise would be easier with an under-inflated ball, this is not so.

DUMBBELL FLY

Primary Muscles Worked: Pectoralis major, anterior deltoid

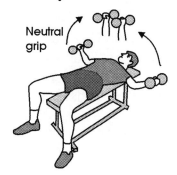

Neutral grip

Quick Tip: Halt the eccentric phase when the elbows are at the level of the shoulders.

Exercise Technique: Obtain two dumbbells of equal weight and lay supine on a stable exercise bench. Use a closed grip for the duration of the exercise. Wrists are rigid and not bent during the exercise. Extend arms to a soft lock-out position (slight bend in elbows) with a neutral grip (palms facing each other). The arms should be at or just below shoulder level. In this position the elbows should be pointed outward, away from the body. Eccentric phase: Slowly lower the arms while maintaining a soft lock-out in the elbows. Traditionally, the eccentric phase stops when the elbows are at or slightly above the shoulder line (midline of body) although individual biomechanics will dictate the safe ROM. Concentric phase: Raise the arms back to the starting point in a "hugging motion." Elbows are in soft lockout throughout the exercise. Repeat for the desired number of reps.

Spotting: It is important that both lifter and spotter agree ahead of time on how the dumbbells will be handled at the end of the lift. Will the spotter take them from the lifter's hands? Will the lifter rise up and rest them on his/her thighs? Proper communication between lifter and spotter can reduce injury during this critical period of the exercise. During this exercise, the spotter will be positioned behind the lifter's head and will either be kneeling or be on one bent knee. The spotter watches the plane of motion of the dumbbells as well as the expression and other body cues of the lifter. During the concentric phase of the lift, the spotter keeps his/her hands near the lifter's wrists. It is not necessary to grasp the wrists of the lifter unless the lifter is in imminent danger of dropping the weights. During the eccentric phase, the spotter also keeps his/her hands close to the lifter's wrists and may also alternate by placing his/her hands at shoulder level to signal the lifter not to lower past this point.

Comments & Suggestions: One common error with this exercise is trying to press the weights as if performing a bench press. Another error is over-accentuated elbow flexion. In general the elbow should not be bent more than about 15°-20°. Some research shows that dumbbell flys may not be as effective at strengthening the pectoralis major and anterior deltoids as barbell or dumbbell bench presses.[129] As such, flys should not be used as the primary chest exercise in most cases. The dumbbell fly is somewhat controversial in some circles in that it may contribute to rotator cuff shoulder injury or exacerbate existing rotator cuff issues. This can occur in many exercises in which the arm is abducted from the midline of the body and/or elbows travel past shoulder level. This exercise is probably best used if limited to lighter weights. While the machine version is safer, it also should be limited to those without shoulder problems.

PEC DECK (MACHINE PEC FLY)

Primary Muscles worked: Pectoralis major, anterior deltoid

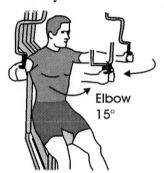

Elbow
15°

Quick Tip: Some versions double as a reverse fly machine. In this case, ensure the handles are properly oriented before using.

Exercise Technique: Adjust the movable arms of the machine so that they are in line with chest (or a little in front of it) when you are sitting in the machine. Sit facing away from the machine. The seat should be adjusted to where the handles are aligned with the nipple line of the chest. Grasp the handles with a closed grip. The elbows should be slightly bent. Wrists should be ridged and not hyper-flexed. Concentric phase: Slowly bring the handles together in a controlled fashion, stopping just before the hands touch. Eccentric phase: Slowly release to starting position and repeat.

Spotting: Trainers should ensure that the seat is at the proper height and that the elbows are slightly bent and do not travel behind the torso during the eccentric phase of the exercise.

Comments & Suggestions. Remind people that many machines of this type can double as a rear delt machine by simply altering the range of motion pins which are usually located near the top of the device. People are often unaware of this and so when they try to use a pec deck that's adjusted to work the rear delts, they have to reach far back to grasp the handles, wrenching their back and shoulders. This can lead to shoulder problems as they perform the exercise with exaggerated ROMs. Remind people also that greater ROM does not always mean greater chest development. Some variations of this machine call for the lifter to place his/her forearms on pads. If this is the case, it is still important to ensure that the elbows do not travel past the torso.

REAR DELT MACHINE/ REVERSE FLY

Primary Muscles Worked: Posterior deltoids, latissimus dorsi, rhomboids.

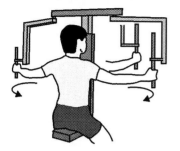

Quick Tip: Pull the shoulder blades together prior to starting this exercise.

Exercise Technique: If this is a piece of equipment that can double as a pec fly, adjust the machine to work the rear delts and sit facing the machine. The chest should be against the pad. Adjust the seat such that the handles are at chest height. Grasp handles and retract shoulder blades. Concentric phase: While keeping a slight bend in the elbows, slowly bring the arms back and outward from the body. Stop when the elbows are in line with shoulders. Eccentric phase: Slowly return the arms to the starting position. Stop just before the weights touch the weight stack. Repeat for desired number of reps.

Spotting: Make sure that the shoulder blades are retracted and that the elbows do not travel past the torso. The lifter's chest should not come off the chest pad. Doing so is cheating and might mean the weight is too heavy. The lifter should not turn his/her head but rather should look straight ahead.

Comments & Suggestions: Since the rear deltoids are often used during lat pull downs, seated rows and other back exercises, it's a personal decision whether to incorporate this exercise. Those performing this movement often force their arms as far back as possible which might place too much stress on the shoulders. This exercise can also be performed with dumbbells or exercise tubing.

PRONE REVERSE FLY WITH STABILTY BALL

Primary Muscles Used: Posterior deltoids, latissimus dorsi, rhomboids, rotator cuff.

Thumb up

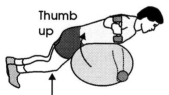

Quick Tip: This can also be performed on a bench if a stability ball is not available.

Exercise Technique: Obtain two light and equal weighted dumbbells and lay prone on a stability ball with the ball at the naval. The legs are extended about hip to shoulder width apart with a slight bend at the knees. The head is neutral and the abs contracted. The exercise is begun with the arms extended outward from the body (maintain a slight bend at the elbows) below the plane of the torso. The hands are oriented such that the thumbs are pointed up (in some variations, this is performed with hands in pronated position). Concentric phase: Slowly, raise the arms upward while keeping the shoulder blades pulled together. Stop when the arms are about shoulder height. Eccentric phase: Slowly return arms to starting position. Repeat.

Spotting: The head stays neutral. The shoulder blades remain contracted. The trunk does not round forward over the ball.

Comments & Suggestions: This is a good rear deltoid exercise and goes well with external rotations and other movements designed to strengthen the rotator cuff. This exercise can also be performed without dumbbells. In this instance, the thumbs should point up to the ceiling. An easier, albeit equally effective, version of this exercise is performed with knees bent and on the floor.

LAT PULL DOWN

Primary Muscles Worked: Latissimus dorsi, posterior deltoid, rhomboids, teres major, trapezius.

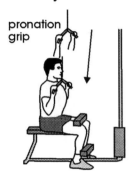

pronation grip

> **Quick Tip:** Pull the shoulder blades together prior to pulling the bar downward.

Exercise Technique: Sit facing the lat pull down machine and grasp the bar with over handed grip (pronated grip). Hand placement on the bar will vary according to individual biomechanics and current/previous injuries, but in general the hands are at shoulder width apart or a little wider. There should be a slight bend in the elbows and the elbows are pointed outward. Lean back slightly (15° - 45°). Retract shoulder blades. Concentric phase: Slowly pull the bar downward to the front of the head. Stop when the upper arms are about parallel with the floor. Hold for a second. Eccentric phase: Slowly let the bar rise to the starting position and repeat. Do not let the bar go so high that the elbows lock out. Always maintain slight bend in elbows. Repeat for the desired number of reps.

Spotting: The spotter stands behind the lifter and makes sure that the lifter is performing the exercise correctly. During heavy lifts, retract shoulder blades. With lighter lifts, holding the retraction may not be needed. A good teaching cue for retraction is to have the person imagine having an ice cube dropped down his/her back. Alternatively, place your finger/fingers between their shoulder blades and have them try to pinch them together. Slightly leaning back (15° -45°) is ok although excessive lean is not. Likewise, rocking back and forth with each rep is considered cheating and may increase injury.

Comments & Suggestions: Pulling the bar behind the head is controversial among many fitness professionals/physical therapists in that some believe it may increase the risk of shoulder injury.[140] Doing so may also strain the cervical neck or injure it if the bar impacts the neck during an overly forceful concentric phase. As divisive as this issue is, few statistics are available to gauge how harmful to the shoulders this movement really is. That being said, it is generally felt that pulling to the front is a safer alternative. Some lifter's may wish to sit facing away from the machine and pull the bar behind the head. This, they often say, places less stress on the shoulder joint. However, sitting straight up does not optimally challenge the latissimus dorsi muscle fibers. Lifter's sometimes advocate using a very wide grip to target the "outer lats." However, there is no such thing as *outer or inner lats*. What very wide grips may do is limit ROM and place greater stress on the shoulder joint which might increase shoulder injury issues. A variation of this exercise is to only retract the shoulder blades without pulling downward with the arms. Doing this also works many of the same muscle groups and often allows more weight to be lifted.

SEATED ROW MACHINE

Primary Muscles Worked: Latissimus dorsi, rhomboids, trapezius, posterior deltoids.

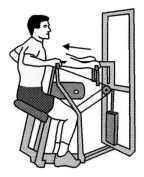

> **Quick Tip:** Retract shoulder blades prior to pulling weight back.

Exercise Technique: Adjust the seat of the machine so that the chest is against the chest pad when seated and the arms are about parallel with the floor. If the machine has an adjustable chest pad, adjust it so that the lifter can reach the handles comfortably yet still have a slight bend in the elbows. Concentric phase: Grasp handles with neutral grip. Retract shoulder blades and pull backward until upper arm is about perpendicular to the floor. Hold for a second. Eccentric phase: Slowly return to the starting position while maintaining shoulder retraction. Repeat for desired number of reps.

Spotting: Stand behind the lifter and place your finger between his/her shoulder blades to prompt them into retraction. Have him/her imagine what they would do if you suddenly dropped an ice cube down their back. Avoid rocking back and forth during the movement. If the shoulders roll forward, it's a sign the weight may be too heavy or the lifter is not holding shoulder blades together.

Comments & Suggestions: On many pulling exercises, we advise lifter's to retract their shoulders blades and hold the retraction throughout the movement. But is this always best? Generally, for heavier loads, yes, because it offers better trunk and shoulder stabilization. For lighter loads, though, (e.g., 15 or more reps) holding the retraction may not be as important. In this situation, retracting and releasing the shoulder blades after each rep offers variety to the exercise. People may also perform this exercise on a seated pulley machine where the torso is not stabilized. If performed in this manner, rocking back and forth is not necessary and may strain the low back. Rather, maintain the torso in an upright posture throughout the exercise. A variation of the seated row is to only retract the shoulder blades without pulling back with the arms. Doing this also works many of the same muscle groups and often allows for more weight to be lifted. It also is a good shoulder stabilizing exercise. The neutral grip is usually preferable to a pronated grip for those with shoulder injuries.

DUMBBELL ONE ARM BENT OVER ROW

Primary Muscles Worked: Posterior deltoids, latissimus dorsi, rhomboids, teres major.

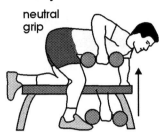

neutral grip

Quick Tip: Remember to retract the shoulder blade. The head should be neutral.

Exercise Technique: Obtain a dumbbell and place on the floor close to the front of a stable exercise bench. Place one knee on the exercise bench (the lower leg will also rest on the bench). The other foot is on the floor, pointed straight ahead with knee slightly bent. The hand which will not grasp the dumbbell is placed on the front or side of the exercise bench for stability. At this point the trunk will be about parallel with the bench. The body weight should be evenly distributed between the bent knee and hand. The head should be neutral, neither looking up or to the sides. Grasp the dumbbell with a neutral grip. Abs should be contracted slightly. Concentric phase: With the dumbbell in line with the shoulders, retract the shoulder blade and slowly pull the dumbbell upward until a 90° bend at the elbow is reached (at this point the upper arm is parallel with the floor). Eccentric phase: Slowly lower the dumbbell to the starting position while maintaining retraction of the shoulder blade. Do not lock out the elbow at the bottom of the eccentric phase. The dumbbell should stay close to the body at all times. Repeat for the desired number of reps.

Spotting: People often twist the trunk in the direction of the pull in an attempt to help them lift the weight. This is cheating due to lifting too much weight. Rather, the chest should be facing down toward the floor. The head should stay neutral, neither looking upward or to the sides.

Comments & Suggestions: While a flat bench is shown here, an adjustable bench elevated to about 30° can also be used. The knee and hand used for support should both be from the same side of the body. That is, if the left knee is bent, stabilize with the left hand and vice versa. For variety, this exercise can also be performed using an exercise ball, a selectorized machine or with exercise tubing. This exercise may aggravate those with carpal tunnel syndrome because of the stress placed on the supporting hand.

MACHINE SHOULDER PRESS

Primary Muscles Worked: Anterior and medial deltoids, triceps, trapezius.

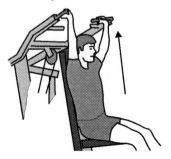

Quick Tip: Grasping the handles with palms facing each other reduces the stress on the shoulders and reduces possible injury.

Exercise Technique: In most versions of this exercise, the person sits facing away from the machine with feet on the floor, about hip width apart. The seat should be adjusted so that the thighs are about parallel with the floor. In the starting position, the elbows should be about shoulder height or a little lower. This may require reducing the seat height. The shoulders are weaker (due to less overlap between actin and myosin protein filaments) when the elbows are lower than shoulder height. This may limit the amount of weight lifted. When the handles are grasped with a closed, pronated grip, the elbows should be pointing out from the sides of the body. The wrists are rigid and not bent backward. Concentric phase: Press upward until soft lockout is reached. Eccentric phase: Slowly lower until elbows are at shoulder height. Repeat for the desired number of repetitions.

Spotting: Common errors during this exercise include excessive arching of the low back, hands too far apart (may be unavoidable with machines), turning the head during the lift and not keeping feet on the floor.

Comments & Suggestions: The shoulder press is sometimes considered controversial because few ADLs involve lifting heavy loads above the head. Use caution with this exercise if the lifter has any neck, shoulder or elbow injuries. If performed with a barbell, some people may lower the bar behind the head. In theory, performing the exercise this way may result in rotator cuff injuries. Pushing from the front of the head is usually deemed the safer way to do this exercise. Many shoulder press machines allow this exercise to be performed with a neutral grip (i.e., palms of hands facing each other), which is usually considered safer for the shoulders.

Spotting: 12 Steps to Success

1. Ask the person how he/she wants to be spotted. Some people have different preferences.
2. Ask the person how many reps he/she can safely perform.
3. Ask the person at what rep he/she thinks they may need help.
4. Ask the person if they need a lift off (i.e., assistance starting the set).
5. Ask the person if he/she want verbal help during the set (e.g., "It's all you, man!").
6. Keep your focus fixed on the lifter at all times.
7. Avoid, if possible, yanking the weight up if you think the lifter can't lift the weight. This may lead to injury.
8. If you've been working out also, make sure you don't drip your own sweat on the lifter while he/she are performing the set.
9. If spotting dumbbell exercises, alternate hand placement between elbows and alongside wrists. Don't just push up on the elbows as this can lead to injury.
10. When handing dumbbells to a lifter, grasp the dumbbells at the ends and hand them to the lifter one at a time. Never grasp dumbbells by the handles when giving them to the lifter.
11. Be willing to say *no* if the lifter is using more weight than you feel comfortable handling.
12. With heavy squats, two spotters —one at each end of the bar — is better than one.

LATERAL RAISE WITH DUMBELLS

Primary Muscles Worked: medial deltoids.

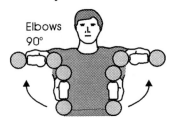

Elbows 90°

Quick Tip: The elbows should go no higher than the shoulders.

Exercise Technique: Grasp two equal weight dumbbells and stand with arms bent at 90°. The palms should be facing each other (neutral grip). If performed standing, the feet should be about hip-shoulder width apart. Slightly lean forward at hips. Concentric phase: Slowly raise the dumbbells until the elbows are at the height of the shoulders. Eccentric phase: Slowly lower dumbbells to the starting position.

Spotting: Make sure the elbows do not travel higher than the shoulders as this may increase shoulder problems or exacerbate existing shoulder problems.

Comments & Suggestions: This exercise can be performed either seated or standing. Typically, this exercise is performed with arms extended outward to the sides of the body. If doing this version remember to keep a slight bend in the elbows. The exercise shown here is a modified version which takes stress off the elbows. Because the shoulder is not very strong in this position, it's not necessary to use heavy weights. Gyms typically have machines for this exercise. If using a machine, raise the seat height until the shoulders are in line with the rotational points of the machine. On newer machines, this is often highlighted by a colored plastic cover or sticker. Also, with machines, try not to grasp the handles too much as this is cheating. Let the shoulders do the lifting. This exercise may exacerbate rotator cuff injuries. A safer alternative to the lateral raise is *scaption* whereby the lifter holds a light weight (or resistance band) with arms at the sides but slightly forward (~30°) and thumbs pointing up. In this position, raise the straightened arms (soft lockout at elbow) up until they are about shoulder height and lower to starting position.

The Rotator Cuff

Because of its great ROM, the shoulder is very prone to injury. One common injury is to the rotator cuff. The rotator cuff represents four muscles that keep the upper arm bone (humerus) in its socket (glenoid fossa) and is very active during all shoulder exercises. The muscles of the rotator cuff are the supraspinatus, infraspinatus, subscapularis and teres minor. Rotator cuff injuries are common in baseball, tennis, basketball, weightlifting, swimming or any activity where the arms are regularly raised over the head.

Common signs include shoulder pain especially when reaching over the head or when lifting weights (e.g., bench pressing, push-ups or shoulder press) or when reaching the arm behind the back. Sometimes the pain occurs when not moving and may even cause almost total lack of mobility in the arm. In extreme cases there may be a tear of the rotator cuff muscles which may require surgery. Usual treatment includes ice to relive inflammation, resting the area and halting the activity which caused the injury. A physician may inject steroids (e.g., cortisone) into the area, prescribe pain relievers and refer the person to a physical therapist who can recommend various exercises (e.g., external shoulder rotation) to help strengthen the rotator cuff. Rotator cuff exercises are one of the hallmarks of not only helping preventing rotator cuff injuries but also their reoccurrence.

UPRIGHT ROW

Primary Muscles Worked: Anterior, medial and posterior deltoids, trapezius, serratus anterior, brachialis, brachioradialis, biceps.

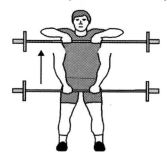

> **Quick Tip:** A wider grip may place less stress on the wrists and rotator cuff.

Exercise Technique: Stand erect and grasp an equal weighted barbell. The knees are slightly flexed, abs contracted with hands pronated and closed around the barbell. Feet should be shoulder width apart. The lifter should be looking straight ahead. The back should be in a neutral position as opposed to "straight." Concentric phase: Pull the bar slowly upward, keeping the bar close to the body at all times. Halt the exercise when the elbows are at the height of the shoulders. Avoid shrugging the shoulders during the exercise. Likewise, do not rise up on toes. Eccentric phase: Slowly lower the barbell until the arms are almost fully extended. Keep the bar close to the body at all time. Repeat for the desired number of repetitions.

Spotting: Make sure the knees are slightly bent, and that the elbows do not rise above shoulder height (doing so may increase shoulder injuries). Ensure that the head does not turn to the sides.

Comments & Suggestions: The upright row is controversial in some circles in that it may increase the risk of shoulder injuries (e.g., osteoarthritis, bursitis, rotator cuff injuries). As such, many trainers and physical therapists don't recommend it. During the concentric phase, the humorous may pinch the tendons of the rotator cuff which may result in *impingement syndrome*. As such, people with shoulder impingement syndrome (or any shoulder issue) may want to avoid this movement. Traditionally, the upright row is performed with the hands close together on the bar. In theory, this may place excessive forces on the wrists. Some modify this exercise by using dumbbells or by holding the hands shoulder width apart in the hopes of reducing shoulder and wrist injury. Another modification is to lift the elbows to shoulder height and no higher.

Controversial Exercises

Exercise	Reason
Upright rows	Possible increased risk of shoulder problems
Behind head military press	Possible increased risk of shoulder problems
Behind head lat pull down	Possible increased risk of shoulder problems
Good Mornings	Possible increased risk of low back problems
Deep knee squats (>90°)	Possible increased risk of knee problems

EXTERNAL SHOULDER ROTATION WITH DUMBBELL

Primary Muscles Worked: Rotator Cuff Muscles (primarily infraspinatus and teres minor).

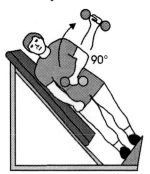

> **Quick Tip:** For added difficulty, perform on the floor.

Exercise Technique: Obtain a light dumbbell and lie on your side, on a stable incline exercise board (or floor or flat bench for added difficulty). The arm to be used should be bent at 90°. A towel can be used under the head for comfort if desired. Concentric phase: Rotate the bent arm outward from the body, stopping close to the end of pain-free normal ROM or if the elbow moves away from the body. Eccentric phase: Slowly lower to the starting position and repeat.

Spotting: A common error is moving the elbow away from the body. Having the lifter hold a towel between the elbow and torso should eliminate this from occurring. Alternately, the spotter may place one or two fingers on the elbow to remind the lifter of the proper position.

Comments & Suggestions: People are usually stronger doing *internal shoulder rotation* than external rotation. Thus, an imbalance between these muscles might contribute to shoulder instability. For this reason, external shoulder rotation should be a staple in all exercise programs. Rotator cuff injuries are common in many sports (e.g., tennis, golf, baseball pitchers). There are several variations of this exercise. The version shown in the picture is less intense than that usually performed (on the floor). The exercise can also be performed standing, using elastic tubing. The exercise can also be performed with no equipment by having the person's opposing hand provide resistance while external rotation is performed. Normally, external and internal rotations are performed with lighter resistances and higher number of reps (e.g., 15-20 reps).

SHOULDER FLEXION WITH DUMBBELLS

Primary Muscles Worked: Anterior deltoid, pectoralis major.

Neutral
grip

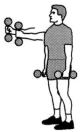

> **Quick Tip:** Performing with exercise tubing or a cable machine may strengthen the muscles over a greater ROM than dumbbells.

Exercise Technique: Obtain two equal weighted dumbbells and stand with feet shoulder width apart with a slight bend in the knees and hips. The dumbbells should be at sides, held with neutral grip. There should be a slight bend in the elbows at all times. Concentric phase: Slowly raise dumbbells up and in front of the body while maintaining a slight bend at the elbows. Stop when hands are at about shoulder level (i.e., parallel with floor). Eccentric phase: Slowly lower to starting position. Repeat for desired number of reps.

Spotting: The lifter should look straight ahead and not turn his/her head to sides. The dumbbells should not tilt down at the wrists. This occurrence may signify that the weight is too heavy for the lifter.

Comments & Suggestions: This exercise is also known as the front raise or front deltoid raise. Some lifter's perform this exercise with a pronated (palms down) grip, which reduces the influence of the biceps muscles. Because the shoulder is relatively easy to injure and because this is a single joint exercise, work at higher numbers of reps (e.g., 15 reps) and keep the weight light. This exercise can also be performed seated or with exercise tubing or a cable machine.

Basic Shoulder Safety Guidelines

Warm up first	Stop if any sharp pain is felt
Maintain strength in rotator cuff	Use proper form
Avoid pressing behind the head	Don't lift more than you can safely handle
Avoid pulling the lat bar behind the head	Don't let elbows travel past torso (e.g., flys)

BARBELL SHRUG

Primary Muscles Worked: Upper trapezius, rhomboids, levator scapulae.

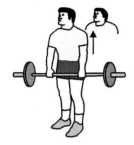

Quick Tip: Remember to keep a slight bend at the knees during this movement.

Exercise Technique: Hold an equal weighted barbell in front of the body (it can also be held behind the body as well). Hands are pronated and should be held a little wider than shoulder width apart. Elbows are slightly bent. There should be a slight bend in the knees. The lifter will now have a slight forward lean which is ok. Concentric phase: Slowly raise the shoulders upward. In this position, the shoulders will travel slightly behind the neck. This is ok. Eccentric phase: Slowly lower the barbell to the starting point while maintaining a slight bend at the elbows. Repeat for desired number of repetitions.

Spotting: The lifter's head should look straight ahead and not turn. There should be a small bend in the knees and the lifter should be slightly leaning forward which helps to better recruit the muscles used.

Comments & Suggestions: This exercise can also be performed with dumbbells which can either be held at the sides or in front of the body. Regardless of which variation is used, it is not necessary to roll the shoulders while performing this exercise. Doing so is unnecessary because it works the muscles perpendicular to gravity, which does not effectively work the muscles.

SUPINE LEG PRESS MACHINE

Primary Muscles Worked: Quadriceps (vastus lateralis, vastus medialis, vastus intermedius, rectus femoris), hamstrings (semimembranosus, semitendinosus, biceps femoris), gluteal muscles.

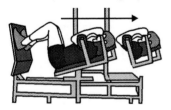

Quick Tip: Make sure toes are at least as high as knees.

Exercise Technique: Adjust the machine to the appropriate weight and recline with shoulders under the pads and feet on the metal platform. Feet should be at hip width apart with toes at least as high as knees if not a little higher. Concentric phase: Press feet into the foot plate, lifting the weight stack and halting just before full knee lock out occurs (i.e., perform a soft lock out). Eccentric phase: Slowly lower the weight stack, halting just before the weights touch.

Repeat for the desired number of reps.

Spotting: Ensure that the lifter's feet are at least as high as his/her knees and that the back is not arching. The spotter also reminds the lifter to breathe during the activity.

Comments & Suggestions: The supine leg press is one of several variations of this exercise. All basically challenge the same muscle groups similarly. Other popular types include the 45 degree leg sled and seated leg press. One of the most common leg press mistakes is performing the exercise with the knees placed higher than (i.e. in front of) the toes. Doing so places perpendicular forces (sheering forces) on the knees and can increase pain. Another common mistake is letting the knees bow inward during the lift. The knees should be at about hip or shoulder width apart during the lift. Arching of the low back may occur on the supine leg press when the lifter attempts to lift more weight than he/she can handle. If this occurs, it may be prudent to reduce the resistance and lift that load slower or alternatively, move to another type of leg exercise Some versions have a low back support to help reduce arching of the low back.

Leg Press vs. Squat

The leg press is often said to be a safer alternative to the squat performed with free weights. This point is debatable and really depends on the person we are talking about. The squat is more sport-specific than the leg press. That is to say, athletics do not usually only involve leg strength but also balance and strength of the entire core musculature. Because they tend to stabilize the low back and core, only performing leg presses in theory, might increase the risk of injury in athletes. One might also make this point with the general population as well, given that many daily tasks require an integrated effort of the body as a whole rather than simply the legs. Conversely, it's generally easier to make lifting mistakes with the squat. Regardless, the real definition of which is safer depends on the person's unique health history and/or goals. For those with back injuries or balance issues, the leg press might be safer. For novices, it's probably best to start by teaching the leg press and progress to the squat over time.

SQUAT (WITH STABILITY BALL)

Primary Muscles Used: Quadriceps (vastus lateralis, vastus medialis, vastus intermedius, rectus femoris), hamstrings (semimembranosus, semitendinosus, biceps femoris), gluteal muscles, calves.

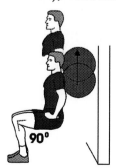

Quick Tip: For added difficulty, use dumbbells and/or combine with biceps curl, lateral raise or shoulder press.

Exercise Technique: Obtain a properly inflated stability ball and place against a wall. Prior to the exercise, the ball should be positioned at about the lower back region. Feet should be about shoulder width apart with toes pointing straight ahead. There should be a slight bend in the knees. Eccentric phase: Slowly lower the body (as if sitting down in a chair), being mindful not to increase the lean of the torso during the descent nor to let the knees travel past the toes. Descend to approximately 60° to 90° or to where comfortable. Concentric phase: Slowly rise up to starting position, halting the movement just before knees lock out. Repeat for the desired number of reps.

Spotting: Ensure that the knees don't travel in front of the toes when viewed from the side. If the knees do, bring the feet further out from the wall and/or instruct the person to "push your butt into the wall."

Comments & Suggestions: Make sure the person can do a wall squat and/or has sufficient balance before introducing the stability ball. For added difficulty, dumbbells, elastic tubing, or other forms of resistance may be used. Pressing up through the heels places more stress on the glutes. If performing in the home, be aware that eventually the ball may leave a mark on the walls.

SQUAT (WITH DUMBBELLS)

Primary Muscles Used: Quadriceps (vastus lateralis, vastus medialis, vastus intermedius, rectus femoris), hamstrings (semimembranosus, semitendinosus, biceps femoris), gluteal muscles, calves.

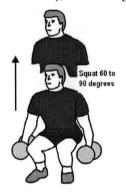

Squat 60 to 90 degrees

Quick Tip: For added difficulty, perform while sitting down on a bench and/or rest dumbbells vertically on shoulders.

Exercise Technique: Obtain two equal weighted dumbbells and hold at sides with neutral grip. Feet should be about shoulder width apart with toes pointing straight ahead. There should be a slight bend in the knees. Eccentric phase: Slowly lower the body (as if sitting down in a chair), being mindful not to let the knees travel past the toes. Descend to approximately 60° to 90° or to where comfortable. Concentric phase: Slowly rise up to starting position, halting the movement just before the knees lock out. Repeat for the desired number of reps.

Spotting: Ensure that the knees don't travel in front of the toes when viewed from the side and that the heels do not come off the floor during the exercise. Also check whether the torso is flexing forward too much. This can enhance stress on the low back. The lifter should look straight ahead, not up to the ceiling. Knees should not lock out at the top of the movement.

Comments & Suggestions: It's better to look straight ahead rather than look up to the ceiling during squats as this will help the lifter maintain balance. It is often said to keep the back "straight". Technically this is incorrect because there is a natural curve in the human spinal cord. Instead, keep the back in a neutral position. Remember that inflexibility can limit ROM in the squat. Beginners usually squat wrong, pushing the knees past the toes. The often-recited advice of "pushing with the heels," which emphasizes the glutes more, may cause novices to lose balance and fall backward. Alternatively, try distributing the weight evenly over the feet. It is usually recommended not to squat below 90° (i.e., where thighs are parallel with floor) because once past this point, the stress on the knees increases dramatically. In theory, this may enhance/promote knee problems/pain. Dumbbell placement alters the feel of this exercise (e.g., dumbbells on shoulders vs. held at sides) and makes for good variations in this movement. This exercise can also be performed using a stability ball placed against a wall.

SQUAT WITH BARBELL

Primary Muscles Used: Quadriceps (vastus lateralis, vastus medialis, vastus intermedius, rectus femoris), hamstrings (semimembranosus, semitendinosus, biceps femoris), gluteal muscles.

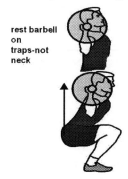

rest barbell on traps-not neck

Quick Tip: Don't let knees go past toes. Look straight ahead— not upward to the ceiling.

Exercise Technique: Load an equally weighted barbell onto a power rack that has been adjusted to be at shoulder height or a little lower (this will allow the lifter to pick up and re-rack the weight easier). Stand under the bar with feet about shoulder or hip width apart and pointed straight ahead. The bar should rest on the upper back and posterior deltoids near the trapezius and be grasped a little wider than shoulder width with a closed pronated grip. In this position, the elbows are pointed outward from and behind the body to help keep the weight on the upper back. The weight should be evenly distributed over this area. Pull shoulder blades together. The head looks straight ahead (not up to the ceiling). Now, lift the weight upward by extending at the hips and knees. The barbell is now resting freely on the upper body. Take a step or two backward in preparation for the eccentric phase of the lift. Feet are still about shoulder to hip width apart and pointed straight ahead. Eccentric phase: Flex at the hips and knees and slowly lower the body, remembering not to lean too far forward. Stop the decent when about 60°-90° of knee flexion is reached (at 90° the thighs will be about parallel with the floor). Hold for a second. Concentric phase: Extend at the hips and knees (as getting up from a chair) to a standing position, being conscious not to lock out the knees at the top of the movement. Repeat for the desired number of reps.

Spotting: Ensure the knees do not shoot past the toes and that the lifter does not descend lower than 90° or where he/she feels comfortable. If the heels come off the floor, the lifter has gone too low for their level of flexibility. The knees should remain the same distance apart during the lift and should not bow inward or outward. Technically, at least two people should spot the squat —one on each end of the bar. This way, each spotter can cup their hands together and grasp the end of the barbell to easily help with lift-offs or if the lifter needs assistance.

Comments & Suggestions: The technique described here is different than for powerlifting and other competitive weightlifting events where squatting lower than 90° may be necessary. Lower body flexibility impacts the ability to perform the squat. Inflexibility in the lower body can contribute to the compression forces felt on the spine. Placing blocks or weight plates under the heels can increase the stress on the knees.

Common Squat Mistakes

Mistake	Reason
Sacrificing form for weight lifted	Greatly enhances overall injury risk
Squatting below 90°	In theory, may increase injury to knee joints
Resting barbell on cervical spine	Weight might fracture cervical spinal bones
Bouncing at bottom of exercise	Increases stress on knee joints and low back
Performing lifts too fast	Increases the overall injury risk potential
Knees traveling past toes	In theory, increases injury to knee joints
Lifting too much weight	May activate GTO and muscle spindles resulting in muscles relaxing when they are not supposed to. May increase injury due poor technique and overloading muscles before they are ready.
Looking upward to the ceiling	May cause neck strain or a loss of balance
Leaning too far forward	May cause loss of balance or neck injury
Toes turning inward	May lead to knee joint injury
Locking out knees	May lead to knee joint injury
Knees bowing inward	May lead to knee joint injury
Uneven gripping of barbell	May lead to loss of balance
Uneven placement of barbell	May lead to loss of balance
Heels coming off the ground	May lead to loss of balance
Bar placed too low on back	May increase stress on shoulders and increase chance of barbell rolling off back
Descending too fast	Lifter misses the advantages of eccentric muscle actions
Hands not pushing up on barbell	Increases risk that bar will slide off back

LUNGE (WITH DUMBBELLS)

Primary Muscles Used: Quadriceps (vastus lateralis, vastus medialis, vastus intermedius, rectus femoris), hamstrings (semimembranosus, semitendinosus, biceps femoris), gluteal muscles, calves (gastrocnemius, soleus).

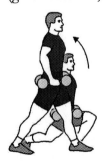

> **Quick Tip:** Don't let knee travel in front of toes. Perform without dumbbells first.

Exercise Technique: Stand upright with weight evenly positioned over feet. Feet should be about hip width apart and pointing straight ahead. Hold equally weighted dumbbells with neutral grip (palms facing in). Eccentric phase: While keeping dumbbells close to body, step forward to where there is no more than a 90° bend at the knee (when thigh is parallel with floor). Remember, 90° may be too far for some. The lifter's competency, balance, leg strength and flexibility will dictate how far he/she can step forward with this exercise. The knee should not move from side to side but stay in the same plane. Concentric phase. Press the extended foot into the floor to lift the body back to the starting position. Advanced lifter's may be instructed to "press through the heel" as this may place more stress on the gluteal muscles. Repeat for the desired number of reps.

Spotting: Ensure that the forward knee does not travel in front of toes and the shoulders do not travel past the hips. The lifter looks straight ahead. The trainer may be positioned at the side so that the lifter can hold onto the trainer's arm for added stability when learning this movement.

Comments & Suggestions: Practice with only bodyweight before incorporating added resistances like dumbbells. Be careful not to step too far forward at first, as this can reduce balance. This exercise can also be performed with a barbell or dumbbells placed at various positions to alter difficulty of exercise. If a barbell is used, make sure it does not rest on the cervical spine. A variation of this exercise calls for the lifter to step backward (sometimes called a reverse lunge).

MACHINE SEATED LEG EXTENSION

Primary Muscles Used: Quadriceps (vastus lateralis, vastus medialis, vastus intermedius, rectus femoris.

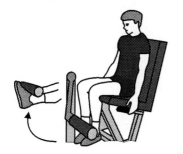

> **Quick Tip:** Align knee with rotational axis of machine.

Exercise Technique: First adjust the machine so that knees are aligned with the axis of rotation and that the leg pads are positioned above the ankles. This usually requires adjusting the seat. Concentric phase: Slowly raise legs as high as comfortable or until soft-lock out. Do not fully lock out knees. Eccentric phase: Slowly lower legs to starting position halting just before the weight plates touch the weight stack. Repeat for the desired number of reps.

Spotting: Normally, the machine is adjusted so that the lifter starts when there is a 90° bend at the knees (i.e., thighs about parallel with floor) and that the knees are aligned with the rotational point of the machine. Ensure that the legs do not "lockout" at the top of the ROM. If the butt lifts off the seat during the eccentric phase, the weight is too heavy. The legs should move slowly during both concentric and eccentric phases with no quick, jerky movements. Likewise, the back should not arch up during this movement.

Comments & Suggestions: While this exercise is usually performed with the toes pointed straight ahead, some, albeit controversial, research suggests that turning the toes inward (internally rotating the leg) recruits more of the vastus lateralis and vastus medialias muscles, while pointing the toes outward (externally rotating the leg) places more stress on the rectus femoris.[130] Many perform this exercise with a 90° bend at the knee, although almost any ROM is possible, especially with machines that have adjustable ROM limiters. The lifter's goals, strength and advice from a physical therapist (if applicable) will dictate the ROM of this exercise. Trainers should remember that greater stresses are placed on the knee joint when the leg is extended to full lockout. Thus, the higher one lifts, in theory, the greater the risk of knee injury. As such, a soft lock out is preferred over totally locking out the knees. Because this is a single joint exercise, it's probably wise to do it after lower body multi-joint exercises like leg presses, squats, etc. For added difficulty, perform this exercise using only one leg at a time. If knee pain is felt with this exercise, don't do it and refer to a medical professional for formal diagnosis of the issue.

Chondromalacia Patella

Chondromalacia patella or "runners knee" is a condition where the knee cap is not properly lined up on the thigh bone. The condition can occur following an injury, overuse or no injury. Weakness in the thighs or having flat feet may also contribute to the problem.[138] Common signs include pain behind the knee cap or behind the knee, pain felt walking up or down stairs or after being seated for long periods of time.[133,138] People may also feel sensations of grinding under the knee when they extend their leg. Treatment often includes rest and icing the area as well as stretching the quadriceps, hamstrings and calves. Warming up prior to activity can also help. In addition, strengthening of the quadriceps may also be required. If using a leg extension machine, adjust the machine so that that the leg only lifts up 6-8 inches before full leg extension occurs.[138] Alternatively, sit on the floor with leg to be strengthened extended. Lift the straightened leg about 6-8 inches. Lower and repeat.

MACHINE SEATED HAMSTRING CURL

Primary Muscles Worked: Hamstrings (semimembranosus, semitendinosus, biceps femoris).

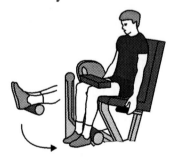

> **Quick Tip:** Align knee with rotational axis of machine.

Exercise Technique: Sit in the machine with legs over the leg pad. There should be a slight (10° to 20°) bend in the knees. If possible, adjust the lower leg pad so that it is positioned at the ankles, just above heels (at Achilles tendon). The heels should be relaxed during the movement. Check to see if the middle/rear aspect of the knees (when viewed from the side) are lined up with the axis of rotation of the machine. If not, adjust the seat. Note: the knees should be lined up with the rotational point through the full ROM. This may require testing with a light resistance first. The thigh support pad (if applicable) should be in contact with thighs (not knees). Concentric phase: Sitting upright in the machine with buttocks pressed into back pad and contract the abs. Now, in a controlled manner, slowly pull the legs downward halting the movement at about 90 ° of knee flexion. At 90 ° the lower legs will be perpendicular to the thighs. Hold contraction for a second. Eccentric phase: Slowly allow the legs to return to their starting position. Stop just before the weight plates of the machine touch. Repeat for the desired number of reps.

Spotting: Make sure the middle part of the knee is aligned with the machine's axis of rotation during the entire ROM. This is easiest seen when kneeling at the side of the machine. The rotation axis can sometimes be identified by a small colored dot or plastic cup that covers or highlights the axis. Make sure the toes do not rotate outward or inward as this may increase stress on the knee.

Comments & Suggestions: Failure of the lifter to sit upright in the machine may be a sign of hamstring inflexibility. Some machines of this type start the ROM with feet higher than knees which puts the knee in a hyper-flexed position, which, in theory, may increase knee injuries. This machine is usually preferable to the prone version for people with heart disease and high blood pressure. Many machines have numbers to help lifter's remember their settings. This can help trainers who design programs for people they see infrequently. This exercise can also be performed with a stability ball for added difficulty.

MACHINE PRONE HAMSTRING CURL

Primary Muscles Worked: Hamstrings (semimembranosus, semitendinosus, biceps femoris).

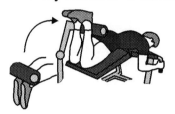

> **Quick Tip:** Align knee with rotational axis of machine. People with heart disease may get dizzy if they rise too fast from this machine.

Exercise Technique: Adjust the weight stack to the desired resistance. Adjust the ankle pad (if possible) so that it rests above the heels. Lay face down (prone) on the machine with the legs under the ankle pad. In this position, the knees should have a slight (10-20°) bend in them. If the machine has hand grips, grasp them lightly. The knees should be slightly off the pad. The knees should also be lined up with the rotational axis of the machine. A small, colored circular dot or plastic cup may highlight this area. The feet are relaxed. Concentric phase: Slowly the lift legs until a 90° bend at the knee is reached (at 90° the ankles will point straight up). Eccentric phase: Slowly lower to starting position, halting just before the weight stack touches the other weight plates. Do not lock out knees at the end of the eccentric phase. Repeat for the desired number of reps.

Spotting: Make sure the hips do not come off the machine. This may stress the low back. Angled benches make this less likely but it may still happen. The knees should be off the edge of the thigh pad, not pressed into the pad. There should be a slight bend at the knees when the legs are extended. The middle part of the knees should be aligned with the rotational axis of the machine. Don't let the lifter's head arch up on this exercise.

Comments & Suggestions: Because more tension is on the hamstrings in the prone position, this exercise may work the hamstrings more than the seated version. By the same token, this movement may be more difficult in those with tight hamstrings. It is not necessary for the ankle pad to touch the buttocks during the concentric phase. People with heart disease and/or blood pressure issues may get dizzy if they rise too fast from this machine due a temporary drop in blood pressure (orthostatic hypotension). This may result in injury if they fall. For those and people with back problems, the seated version may be a safer alternative. For novices, the seated version is probably better if you only see them occasionally.

HAMSTRING CURL WITH STABILITY BALL

Primary Muscles Used: Hamstrings (semimembranosus, semitendinosus, biceps femoris).

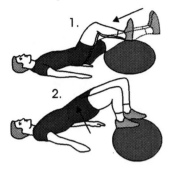

> **Quick Tip:** Keep the buttocks elevated during the exercise. Bringing the arms closer to the sides increases the difficulty.

Exercise Technique: Obtain a stability ball and lie supine on the floor. Extend the legs and place the tops of the heels or ankles on the ball. Extend the arms out to the sides to about 45° to aid with stability. Extend the hips by pressing heels/ankles into the ball and lifting the buttocks off the floor with legs extended (maintain slight bend in the knees). This is the starting position prior to beginning the exercise. Slowly draw the ball toward you by bending at the knees. Hold for a second. Now, move the ball away by extending the legs. Stop when there is a slight bend at the knees. Repeat for the desired number of reps.

Spotting: The hips/buttocks should remain elevated and the body should not wobble while performing the exercise. The head should not come off the floor.

Comments & Suggestions: To learn this movement, it may be necessary to first strengthen the core by performing with calves on ball and only raising the buttocks into air. Because this exercise uses the stability ball, more than the hamstrings are being utilized. Other muscles involved include the calves as well as the abs and back muscles. While keeping the hips elevated is important, it is not necessary to thrust the hips upward as shown in this picture. That is an advanced form of the exercise and can be something to work up to.

SEATED OUTER THIGH MACHINE

Primary Muscles Used: Gluteus medius, gluteus minimus, tensor fasciae latae.

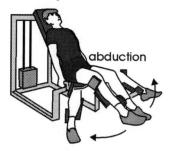

Quick Tip: The outer part of the knee should be lined up with the knee pads.

Exercise Technique: The exercise is started with the legs inside the knee pads and the legs close to each other (this may require an adjustment to the machine). The knee pads should be against the outer part of the knees. In some versions, the knees are bent to 90°. Some versions also have a place to rest the feet during the exercise. Concentric phase: Slowly press against the leg pads and open the legs to a comfortable position (for many, this is about 45°). Hold for a second. Eccentric phase: Slowly lower to starting position, stopping just before the weight stack touches. Repeat.

Spotting: The knees should be about parallel with the floor and in some versions of the machine, bent to about 90°. The low back should not arch during the exercise.

Comments & Suggestions: The technical name for this exercise is *hip abduction* because the hips are moving the hips away (abducting) from the body. Physical therapists and occupational therapists often say "AB-duction" so it's not confused with "ADD-duction" – adding or moving the body part toward the body. Not all machines have a weight stack. In other versions, air resistance, supplied by pistons, may be used. Still other versions combine this exercise with working the inner thighs, such that pressing the knees apart works the outer thigh while pulling the knees together works the inner thigh. It's a myth that this exercise reduces body fat (i.e., saddlebags) from the sides of the hips.

SEATED INNER THIGH MACHINE

Primary Muscles Used: Gracillis, adductor longus, adductor magnus, adductor brevis, pectineus.

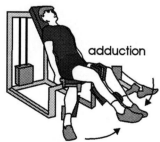

Quick Tip: The inner part of the knees should be lined up with the knee pads.

Exercise Technique: If necessary, first adjust the machine so that the knee pads are close together. Sit in the machine with the inner knees aligned with the knee pads. Rest the feet on the foot supports (if applicable). Now, open the legs to a comfortable position, which for many people is when they feel a slight pull on their inner thighs. If the low back arches, the legs are open too wide.

This is the starting position of the exercise. Concentric phase: Slowly close legs by pressing the knees against the knee pads until the knee pads touch each other. Hold for a second. Eccentric phase: Slowly release the tension, opening the legs to the starting position. Repeat. At the end of the set, readjust the knee pads so that the legs are close together before exiting the machine.

Spotting: The low back should not arch during the exercise. Both concentric and eccentric phases should be performed in a slow, controlled manner. Letting the legs open quickly while under tension may result in injury.

Comments & Suggestions: Adduction (or AD-duction as PTs call it) refers to moving a body part closer (i.e., adding) to the midline of the body. While this exercise can strengthen the inner thigh muscles, it is a myth that it burns fat from the inner thighs. For most people, it's not necessary to open the legs more than about 45° before starting the movement. In some versions of this machine, the legs are bent to 90° during the exercise. This exercise can also be performed by squeezing a stability ball between the legs.

HIP EXTENSION WITH MULTI-HIP MACHINE

Primary Muscles Used: Hamstrings (semimembranosus, semitendoninosus, biceps femoris), gluteus maximus.

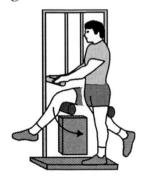

> **Quick Tip:** The upper body should not lean forward or backward during the exercise. That's cheating.

Exercise Technique: Adjust the machine so that the hip is lined up with the rotational point of the machine. Adjust the knee pad so that it is elevated and behind the knee when the leg is raised and flexed as shown in the picture. The other leg is slightly bent at the knee. The hands lightly grasp the stabilizing arm of the machine for support. Concentric phase: Slowly bring the leg backward, halting when it is past the stationary leg (note: how far one presses backward depends on one's ability to stay upright in a neutral position). Eccentric phase: Slowly release tension until the leg is at its starting position. Repeat for the desired number of reps.

Spotting: The upper body should not lean forward or backward during the exercise. The hip should be aligned with the rotational axis of the machine. The head should look forward and not turn to the sides.

Comments & Suggestions: Some versions have an adjustable footplate which helps align the lifter with the rotational point of the machine; while in other versions, the main rotation apparatus can be lowered or raised. In theory, this exercise may exacerbate low back problems in some individuals.

STIFF LEG DEAD LIFT

Primary Muscled Used: Hamstrings (semimembranosus, semitendoninosus, biceps femoris), gluteal muscles, erector spinae.

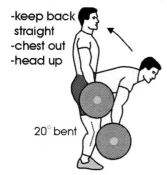

-keep back straight
-chest out
-head up

20° bent

> **Quick Tip:** Keep the weight close to the body and don't lock out the knees.

Exercise Technique: Obtain an equally weighted Olympic bar or barbell and stand over it with feet about shoulder to hip width apart. The feet should be either pointed straight ahead or slightly angled outward. Squat down and grasp the bar with a closed, pronated grip which is about shoulder width apart. In this position, the back should be firm and arched slightly and the chest should be oriented forward and upward (not rounded down). The head is elevated a little bit. Now, pull the shoulder blades together and lift the barbell upward, keeping it close to the body. At the top of the starting point the knees should be slightly flexed (e.g., 20°). Eccentric phase: Slowly lower the barbell by bending at the hips while maintaining the slight bend in the knees. The back stays neutral and rigid and the shoulders are still pinched together and are not rounded forward. The descent stops if the heels come off the floor or when the lifter feels a contraction in the hamstrings. Concentric phase: While still maintaining a slight bend at the knees, extend the hips and slowly ascend to an erect position, keeping the weight close to the body. Repeat for the desired number of reps.

Spotting: It is very important that the weight stay very close to the body at all times. Failure to do so increases injury risk. Ensure that the shoulders don't round forward. In general, the shoulders should not be lower than the hips during the decent phase. Flexing so far that the torso is parallel with the ground greatly increases injury risk. Sometimes lifter's flex at the wrists. This is wrong. The wrists should not bend. No bouncing or exploding upward during the movement should occur as this increases injury. The spine should not hyperextend during the ascent phase.

Comments & Suggestions: Lifers sometimes call stiff leg deadlifts, "stiffies," but this does not mean the knees are stiff, in a locked-out stance. Rather, a slight bend is maintained at the knee during this movement (i.e., soft lockout). This exercise can also be performed with dumbbells, some types of plate-loaded equipment or in the case of beginners, with no weight at all. This is a complicated movement. Bending at the waist, especially when holding an external resistance, places the low back under a lot of stress and greatly enhances the injury risk to the spinal disks of the low back.[132] If performed wrong, this movement can cause injury.[132] Lifter's should have a strong foundation in strength training and have very good flexibility in the hamstrings and back before attempting. This exercise is not for beginners. Some lifter's perform this movement standing on an exercise bench to obtain greater ROM. This further increases injury rate and should not be performed. This movement should not be performed by those with injuries or previous injuries to the low back. Likewise the movement might exacerbate injuries to the knees, neck or shoulders.

DEADLIFT WITH BARBELL

Primary Muscles Worked: Gluteus maximus, hamstrings (semimembranosus, semitendinosus, biceps femoris), erector spinae, quadriceps (vastus lateralis, vastus intermedius, vastus medialias, rectus femoris), rhomboids, trapezius, deltoids.

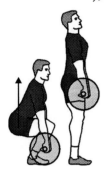

> **Quick Tip:** Keep the weight close to the body at all times.

Exercise Technique: Load an Olympic bar (or barbell) with equal weight on each side. The lifter's feet should be between shoulder and hip width apart and pointed straight ahead (slightly pointed outward is ok also). The lifter squats and grasps the bar with an alternated grip that is slightly wider than shoulder width apart. The back is stiff and rigid. The shoulder blades should be retracted and the chest oriented up. In this position the shoulders will be slightly over the barbell. Concentric phase: Slowly lift the barbell upward by extending the hips and knees (think of standing up from a seated position) while keeping the weight evenly distributed over the feet. The chest is still oriented upward. Continue the lift until standing straight up (with knees slightly flexed). Don't hyperextend the back. The barbell should be close to the body throughout the movement. Eccentric phase: Flex at the hips and knees, lowering the barbell to the floor while at the same time, keeping it close to the body. Touch the floor lightly with the barbell while keeping tension in the muscles as the lifter prepares for the next concentric action. Repeat for the desired number of reps.

Spotting: Ensure the knees don't travel past the toes and that the shoulders don't round forward. The head should be looking straight ahead or slightly upward.

Comments & Suggestions: The deadlift is a complicated movement. As such, lifter's should first develop a good strength base before progressing to this exercise. Sometimes, lifter's will try to *press through the heels* on this exercise as they do with barbell squats. This is incorrect and may result in injury if the lifter falls backward. Rather, the weight should be evenly balanced over the feet. While an alternated grip was used in this example, a pronated grip can also be used. This exercise can also be performed on some plate-loaded and selectorized machines.

Basic Knee Safety Guidelines

Warm up first	Don't lift too much weight
Don't lock out the knees (e.g., squats). Don't let the knees travel past toes (e.g., squats)	Don't bounce at the bottom of the movement (e.g., squats)
Align knees with rotation axis of machine (e.g., leg extension machine)	Don't turn the toes inward
Don't put blocks/weight plates under the heels	Don't let the knees make contact with ground (e.g., lunges)

Basic Low Back Safety Guidelines

Warm up first	Retract shoulder blades with heavy lifts. Don't round shoulders. Keep weight close to body.
Bend and lift with knees/hips — not with the back	Maintain strong abdominals
Maintain flexibility in hamstrings	Maintain flexibility in quadriceps
Maintain strength in low back muscles	Don't arch the back

Functional Isometrics

Recall that isometrics can help increase strength at specific points in a range of motion only. Recall also that many movements have a point where the movement is the most difficult. This is called the *sticking point*. Functional isometrics build upon this, whereby the lifter performs a resistance exercise yet halts the concentric phase at the sticking point. This is accomplished by some immovable, external resistance. At this point, maximal isometric force is applied. For example, if one were performing a deadlift in a power rack, the pins of the rack could be adjusted to the height where the sticking point is reached. When pressed against the pins, the weight can be lifted no higher. At this point, the lifter is performing an isometric action at the sticking point. While not technically a training program, functional isometrics may help improve strength at one's weakest point.

SEATED CALF RAISE

Primary Muscles Used: Soleus (gastrocnemius, to a lesser extent).

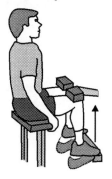

> **Quick Tip:** To avoid injury, determine flexibility in the calves before adding weight to the machine.

Exercise Technique: Sit straight up in the machine with knees bent to 90° and thigh pad just behind the knees resting on the edge of the thighs. In this position the ankles should be perpendicular to the floor. The balls of the feet should be on the raised foot platform. The exercise is started when the calves are supporting the weight to be lifted after it has been removed from its resting location. Concentric phase: Elevate the calves as high as is comfortable. Eccentric phase: Slowly lower the weight until the heels are at least level with the toes or a little below this point. Repeat for desired number of reps.

Spotting: Check that the toes don't slide off the elevated foot platform and that the thigh pad is not compressing the knees. Hand grips are usually present on these machines. The hands should rest comfortably yet not grasp them tightly (this may raise blood pressure) or pull up on them (this is cheating). The knees and toes should stay pointed straight ahead throughout the ROM.

Comments & Suggestions: Both the soleus and gastrocnemius play roles in ankle stability and balance during walking and running as well as most sports. These muscles may also be weak after ACL surgery.[134] The big difference between this exercise and the standing calf raise is that this movement works more of the soleus muscle while the standing calf raise targets more of the gastrocnemius. Because of variations in calf flexibility, it's safest if the trainer assesses how far the heels can lower without any resistance. For example, high-heeled shoes can shorten the Achilles tendon, causing the wearer to have reduced calf flexibility. Sometimes people train calves using a leg press machine. Because in this instance the leg is straightened, the gastrocnemius does more of the work, making it more analogous to a standing calf raise. If no machine is available, this exercise can also be performed seated in a chair with dumbbells resting on the thighs.

Plantar Fasciitis

Plantar fasciitis is a condition characterized by an inflammation of the connective tissue on the bottom of the foot and results in heel pain and stiffness that's usually felt immediately after getting up from being seated for a long time or upon rising from bed. Conditions often linked to this condition include flat feet, tight calves and shoes that have poor arch support. The condition is often seen in those who stand for long periods of time as well as in runners, the overweight and in those who are in poor physical condition. Sometimes increasing the incline on treadmills or walking uphill may make the condition worse as can overtraining/overuse. While exercise can help the condition, calf flexibility is an important part of prevention and treatment. Maintaining flexibility in the calves, using arch supports and/or icing the bottom of the foot if needed can help the condition. Sometimes plantar fasciitis is caused by other conditions that may require referral to a physician or physical therapist.

STANDING CALF RAISE WITH DUMBBELL

Primary Muscles used: Gastrocnemius.

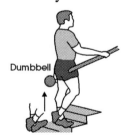
Dumbbell

Quick Tip: Determine how low the heel can go before adding additional weight.

Exercise Technique: Obtain a dumbbell and stand on a step with the balls of the feet at the edge. The dumbbell should be held on the same side as the ankle which is to be worked. The other hand can be used for support. The foot is pointed straight ahead and there is a slight bend at the knee.

Eccentric phase: Slowly lower the heel until tension is felt. Concentric phase: Rise up to the starting position or higher (i.e., plantar flexion), depending on ankle strength. Repeat.

Spotting: The knee should not be locked out. Ensure that the toes do not slide off the step during the movement. The upper body should stay neutral and neither hyperextend backward or flex forward. The head should be neutral and not turn to the sides.

Comments & Suggestions: Both the gastrocnemius and soleus are involved in plantar flexion (raising the heel upward). Together, both muscles form a muscle group that's sometimes called the *triceps surae*. One difference between the two muscles is that the gastrocnemius is made up mostly of type II muscle fibers while the soleus is composed mainly of type I.[135] In this exercise, the gastrocnemius is the main muscle targeted. When seated, the soleus works more. It's safest to first determine flexibility in the calf before adding weight. The normal progression for this movement is to first perform with two feet and no added weight.

Shin Splints

Shin splints are an overuse injury that results in pain felt on the front, inner side of the shins above the ankle. While they can occur in athletes, they tend to be more common in people who are new to exercise and push themselves faster/harder than their bodies can adapt.[138] While any repetitive activity (e.g., jogging) can cause the condition, inadequate warm up and/or stretching prior to activity, using worn out/inappropriate athletic footwear, having flat feet or weak calves can also promote shin splints.[133] Treatment usually consists of rest and icing the area as well as stretching and ankle strengthening exercises. Arch supports may help also. If improvement does not occur after 4 weeks, referral to a physician/physical therapist is warranted.

SPIDER CURLS WITH BARBELL

Primary Muscles Used: Biceps.

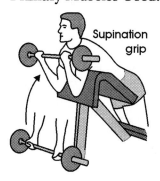
Supination grip

Quick Tip: Pull shoulder blades together and keep the elbows pointed straight ahead.

Exercise Technique: Obtain a barbell and lean against the opposite side of a preacher curl bench. Performed this way, the back of the arms will be against the pad that the chest normally presses against. The hands should be about shoulder width apart. The feet are placed about hip to shoulder width apart and the wrists are neutral and not bent. Pull the shoulder blades together to aid with shoulder stabilization. Eccentric phase: With a closed, supinated grip, slowly lower the barbell until it is almost straight down, (i.e., soft lockout). Concentric phase: Lift barbell until it is between about 90-120°.

Spotting: The head should stay neutral and not become hyperextended. The shoulders should stay neutral and not round forward. The elbows should not flair outward or inward. Hand the barbell to the lifter after he/she gets it to position. Remove barbell when the lifter is finished the set.

Comments & Suggestions: This is a variation of a preacher curl. The advantage here is that it allows the muscle to be worked against gravity over a greater ROM. Some gyms may have benches made specifically for this exercise. Because of the angle, the lifter will probably use less weight than on other biceps exercises. This exercise may exacerbate low back pain in some. This exercise can also be performed with dumbbells or an EZ curl bar. If working out at home, the back of a kitchen chair can also be used.

STANDING BICEPS CURL WITH BARBELL

Primary Muscles Worked: Biceps group, brachioradialis.

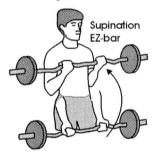
Supination EZ-bar

> **Quick Tip:** Raise the barbell to only 90°. Don't let the elbows drift forward during the exercise.

Exercise Technique: Grasp an equally weighted barbell with a closed, supinated grip. The grip should be at shoulder width apart or a little wider. The knees are slightly bent and the feet are about shoulder to hip width apart. Concentric phase: With the elbows aligned under shoulders, slowly raise the barbell until about it is at about 90° or, if preferred, almost to the height of the shoulders. Eccentric phase: Slowly lower the barbell to the starting position, halting just before the elbows fully lock out. Perform for the desired number of reps.

Spotting: This exercise is usually spotted from behind the lifter so that the trainer can ensure that the elbows do not move from the sides of the body, although spotting from the front is ok also. The lifter's body should not rock back and forth during the exercise. The shoulders should not shrug upward. Ensure also that there is a slight bend in the knees and that the abs are slightly contracted. Make sure the weight is lowered slowly to take full advantage of the eccentric action.

Comments & Suggestions: While an EZ curl bar is shown here, a straight barbell can also be used as well as dumbbells. People often ask which is better for developing the biceps – barbells (straight bar) or an EZ curl bar. While few head-to-head comparisons appear in peer reviewed journals, the straight bar barbell probably out performs the EZ curl bar, in this author's opinion. Anatomically, this has to do with the two functions of the biceps – elbow flexion and supination. By holding the straight bar while curling the barbell (i.e., elbow flexion) one also has his/her hands supinated. By combining both actions of the biceps, one probably puts a greater exercise stress on that muscle.

With the EZ curl bar, the hands are not as supinated. This allows for the other muscles of the arm (brachioradialis and radials) to help. The EZ curl bar, however, does have its place, so performing either of these solely is probably not as good as doing both during one's periodization cycle. Because a barbell is a free weight, it opposes gravity which always acts downward. Because of this, the biceps are maximally contracted (and maximally working against gravity) when the arm is curled to only 90°. Lifting the weight more than this is not wrong, but for those who normally lift through a greater ROM, performing only to 90° will add a nice variety to this exercise. Because the biceps are used in most pulling exercises, a good case can be made that this muscle group is overemphasized in most fitness programs.

MACHINE BICEPS CURL

Primary Muscles Worked: Biceps group, brachioradialis.

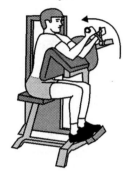

> **Quick Tip:** Align elbows with rotation point of machine.

Exercise Technique: Adjust the seat such that the back of the arms are supported on the arm pads of the machine. The middle portion of the elbows should also be aligned with the rotation point of the machine. This is usually identified by a colored plastic covering or label. Grasp the handles with a closed, supinated grip. The elbows should have a slight bend in them and not be locked out. The chest/upper torso should be against the chest pad of the machine. Concentric phase: Contract biceps and slowly lift until the handles are close to the shoulders or to where it feels comfortable. The wrists should not be bent during the movement. Eccentric phase: Lower the weight in a controlled manner until there is a slight bend in elbows. Repeat for the desired number of reps.

Spotting: The elbows should be aligned with the rotational point of the machine throughout the ROM. The lifter should not rock back and forth or hunch the shoulders as the weight is lifted.

Comments & Suggestions: Some versions of this machine allow the hands to rotate from a pronated (palms facing down) position to a full supination (palms up) position during the ROM. Supination brings the biceps into action more than does pronation. If the exercise is performed with a neutral grip (palms facing each other), the exercise works more of the brachialis and brachioradialis and less biceps. Biceps curls may exacerbate elbow injuries (e.g., tendonitis) in those who have this injury. Use caution in those with osteoporosis; some versions may cause excessive forward trunk flexion that may increase spinal fractures. Because this machine does not rely on gravity for resistance, a greater effective ROM is possible than with free weights. On the downside, this is an isolation exercise that uses less muscle than a standing barbell/dumbbell curl. On some versions of this machine, it's possible to curl the weight up so far that it may impact the head!

STANDING CABLE BICEPS CURL

Primary Muscles Used: Biceps, brachioradialis.

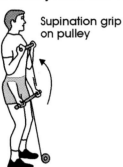

Supination grip
on pulley

> **Quick Tip:** Keep elbows at sides at all times. For a variation, perform while supine on the floor.

Exercise Technique: Stand facing a selectorized cable machine. Grasp handles using a supine, closed grip. The elbows are at the sides and do not move throughout the ROM. The knees are about hip to shoulder width apart and have a slight bend in them. Abs are slightly contracted and the shoulder blades are retracted. Concentric phase: Slowly lift weight stopping at about 90° or a little higher. Eccentric phase: Slowly lower the weight in a controlled manner until there is a slight bend in the elbows. Repeat.

Spotting: Ensure that the upper body does not rock back and forth during the exercise and that the elbows do not move forward, in front of the body. The knees should remain at soft lockout throughout the ROM.

Comments & Suggestions: Because of diversity in design, the same resistance can feel very different between machines. People sometimes try to fight the resistance by bringing the elbows forward, in front of the body. This takes the stress off the biceps and may contribute to tendonitis ("tennis elbow"). Arching of the back is also possible and this, too, should be avoided. This exercise places less stress on the low back if performed supine.

Tennis Elbow

Technically called *lateral epicondylitis*, tennis elbow is one of the most frequent overuse injuries to the elbow. Usually, pain is felt on the outer side (lateral side) of the elbow and results from an inflammation of a tendon. People with tennis elbow frequently report that their elbow hurts when they pick up jars with the arm extended or when they brush their teeth or turn door knobs. Trainers should know this condition does not only happen in tennis players. Any repetitive trauma can cause tennis elbow — including performing too many sets of biceps curls. The biceps muscles tend to be overemphasized in many workout programs. Poor form (i.e., elbows moving forward during the biceps curl) can also contribute to this injury. Treatment usually consists of resting and icing the area followed eventually with gentle stretching and various therapeutic exercises (e.g., reverse wrist curls). Some people may also wear a compression bandage on the upper arm to alleviate the pressure of the tendon pulling on the bone. For acute cases (less than 4 weeks), tennis elbow can usually be resolved within 4-6 weeks; but, if left unchecked for more than two months, the condition may become chronic and it can take up to 6 months before symptoms subside.[133] In the chronic condition, more drastic measures may be required, including steroid injections and physical therapy. In extreme cases, surgery may be required. If the pain is felt on the inner side of the elbow, it is called *medial epicondylitis* or "golfers" elbow.

HAMMER CURL WITH DUMBBELLS

Primary Muscles Worked: Brachialis, brachioradialis.

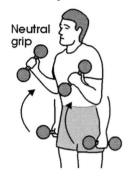

Neutral grip

> **Quick Tip:** For added difficulty, lift dumbbells only to 90°.

Exercise Technique: This exercise can be performed standing or sitting. Grasp two equally weighted dumbbells. The dumbbells should be held in a neutral grip throughout the exercise. Concentric phase. Slowly raise dumbbells to about 90° while keeping the elbows at the sides (at 90° the forearms will be parallel, with the floor). Eccentric phase: Slowly lower to a point just before elbows lock out fully (soft lockout). Repeat for the desired number of reps. If performed standing, the feet should be about hip to shoulder width apart and there should be a slight bend in the knees.

Spotting: This exercise is usually spotted from behind the lifter so that the trainer can ensure that the elbows do not move from the sides of the body, although spotting from the front is ok also. The lifter's body should not rock back and forth during the exercise. The shoulders should not shrug upward. Make certain also that there is a slight bend in the knees and that the abs are contracted. Make sure the weight is lowered slowly to take advantage of the eccentric phase.

Comments & Suggestions: The neutral grip places less emphasis on the biceps group. As a result, this exercise is sometimes overlooked; however, the muscles targeted in this movement can also help with overall biceps development. Remember, there is more to the upper arm than the biceps group. This exercise might be a good alternative for those with wrist problems and may be more functional than biceps curls for people who play sports like tennis.

TRICEPS PUSHDOWN

Primary Muscles Used: Triceps.

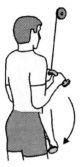

Exercise Technique: Stand facing the machine and grasp the bar with a closed, pronated grip. The grip used can vary from very close (thumbs almost touching each other) to wide (shoulder width apart). The feet should be hip to shoulder width apart. The knees should be slightly flexed and there should be a slight forward lean at the hips, such that the bodyweight is aligned over the ankles. Stand close enough so that the cable hangs straight down when the exercise is performed. Pull the bar down until the arms are bent at about 90° and the elbows are tucked into the sides of the body (i.e., the upper arms are pointed straight down; the forearms are parallel with floor). This is the starting point of the exercise. Concentric phase: Slowly press downward until the arms are almost straight (i.e., soft lock out). Hold for a second. Eccentric phase: Slowly release the tension, which raises the bar back up to the starting position. Repeat for the desired number of reps.

Spotting: A very common mistake is letting the elbows move forward, away from the sides of body. This takes the stress off of the triceps. The elbows may also move backward during the concentric phase. Place towels between the torso and elbows or palpate the lifter's elbows with your fingers so that the elbows remain stationary at the sides of the body. Make sure the hands are evenly spaced on the bar. Two other common mistakes are bending the wrists and turning the head. Rocking back and forth may occur with heavy resistances and should be discouraged.

Comments & Suggestions: Some people perform this exercise standing straight up at attention. At heavier resistances, this practice can put stress to the low back. Bending at the hips and knees reduces this risk. Some cable machines allow this exercise to be performed with one's back pressed against the machine. This better stabilizes the back (good for those with back issues) yet activates the abs to a lesser degree. While a semi-pronated grip is depicted here, a straight bar or a rope can also be used. This exercise can also be performed with dumbbells (i.e., dumbbell kickbacks). If a rope is used, the weight lifted may feel heaver than with a metal bar because the rope is lighter and there is less of a counterweight effect. Because this is a single joint exercise, lifting maximum loads (e.g., 1RM) is not recommended. While a variety of handgrips (supinated, neutral, pronated) can be used with this exercise, none seem to offer any advantage over the other in terms of how much they stimulate the triceps muscles to grow.

TRICEPS EXTENSION MACHINE

Primary Muscles Used: Triceps.

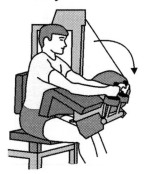

Exercise Technique: Adjust the seat of the machine such that the upper arms are about shoulder height and the elbows are aligned with the rotational point of the machine. The upper arms should be pointing up to the ceiling (i.e., 90° bend at the elbows). The chest should be against the chest pad of the machine (on some versions) and the back in a neutral position (neither hunched forward or hyperextended backward). Concentric phase: Grasp the handles with a neutral grip (palms facing each other) and press forward and downward, halting just before the elbows are completely locked out (i.e., soft lockout). Hold for a second. Eccentric phase: Slowly release the tension, returning to the starting position (i.e., 90° bend at the elbows). Repeat for the desired number of reps.

Spotting: Make certain the elbows are aligned with the axis of rotation of the machine. Neither the elbows nor upper arms should come off the arm pad during the eccentric phase.

Comments & Suggestions: Some versions allow for each arm to be used independently. This can also be performed supine with dumbbells or with a standing triceps pushdown.

TRICEPS KICKBACK WITH DUMBBELL

Primary Muscles Used: Triceps.

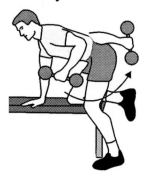

Exercise Technique: Obtain a dumbbell with one hand and place the knee of the opposite side of the body on a stable exercise bench. The dumbbell should be held with a neutral grip during the exercise. Bend forward at the hips and place the other hand on the bench to aid with support. The other leg is on the floor with knee slightly bent. Abs are tight for the entire movement. Generally, the upper torso should be angled slightly upward to about 30°-45° when in this position. Bend the elbow of the hand holding the dumbbell to 90° and hold the upper arm close to the side of the body, making it about parallel with the floor. Concentric phase: Press the dumbbell upward and backward by extending the elbow, while keeping the upper arm stationary at the side of the body. Don't completely lock out the elbow at the top of the movement. Hold for a second. Eccentric phase: Slowly lower to the starting position, stopping when the forearm is pointing straight down. Repeat for desired number of reps.

Spotting: The head should be neutral and the upper torso upward. The wrist should be stationary. If the wrists bend downward, it may signify the weight is too heavy.

Comments & Suggestions: It's not necessary to bring the dumbbell close to the shoulder during the eccentric phase. This engages the brachialis and biceps which are not the target of this exercise. This exercise presents an awkward angle and as such, the weight lifted will be much less than on other triceps exercises. Because triceps are involved in pressing movements they tend to be overemphasized in most exercise programs.

SUPINE TRICEPS EXTENSION WITH DUMBBELLS

Primary Muscles Used: Triceps.

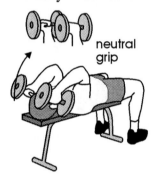
neutral grip

> **Quick Tip:** Upper arms should point upward to ceiling during this movement.

Exercise Technique: Obtain two equally weighted dumbbells and recline supine on a stable exercise bench as shown. The feet should be about hip to shoulder width apart. The exercise is begun with the arms extended (slight bend at the elbows) and dumbbells held over the chest. Eccentric phase: Slowly lower dumbbells toward the forehead or just past it while keeping the upper arms pointed upward to the ceiling. Stop when there is about a 90° bend at the elbows. Concentric phase: Slowly raise dumbbells to starting position, halting just before the elbows lock out. Repeat.

Spotting: The upper arms should be perpendicular to the floor throughout the movement. The low back should not arch upward and the feet should be on the floor. If the back arches, put the feet on a stable box or exercise step. Placement of the feet on the exercise bench is also possible, but this increases the balance requirement of the exercise. Make sure the lifter does not lose their grip on the dumbbells. At no time should the dumbbells make contact with the head.

Comments & Suggestions: This exercise is also called the "skull crusher" because of the possibility of what can happen if the exercise is not performed correctly. Some lifers use a variety of grips when training triceps (e.g., supinated, neutral and pronated). While it does not appear that one grip activates the triceps more than another, altering the grip adds variety and in theory, may reduce overuse injuries. Using a neutral grip may produce less stress on the wrists than a supinated grip, as is often used when performed with a barbell. Moving the upper arms closer to the head (or further away) places the stress on different aspects of the triceps muscle. Many variations exist such as performing while supine on a stability ball and while standing using a rope. This exercise can also be performed using a triceps extension machine.

Triceps Tendonitis

Triceps tendonitis results from an inflammation of the triceps tendon which is located behind the elbow on the upper arm. It can result from overuse (too many chest and triceps exercises) or from overloading the muscles faster than they can adjust.[133] A forceful impact can also cause this condition. Symptoms can include pain, redness and/or warmth over the back of the elbow. Treatment often includes ice, rest, stretching and eventually strengthening of both the triceps and biceps, which work together to keep the elbow structurally sound.[133] If the condition persists for more than two weeks without improvement, a referral to a physician or physical therapist is warranted.

MODIFIED SUPERMAN

Primary Muscles Used: Gluteus maximus, hamstrings, rectus abdominis internal and external obliques, deltoids, rhomboids, trapezius.

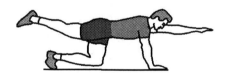

> **Quick Tip:** For added difficulty, try performing while on a stability ball.

Exercise Technique: The exercise is started when the person is supported by having both hands and knees on the floor. Prior to the exercise, the arms should be in line with the shoulders and the knees in line with the hips. The head should be neutral and the trunk should also be neutral, being about parallel with the floor. The abs should be slightly contracted. Performing the exercise: simultaneously raise the right arm and left leg slowly until they are at about trunk level. Hold for 1-2 seconds and lower to starting position. Now, lift the left arm and right leg until they are level with the trunk. Lower to starting position. Alternate the limbs like this for the desired number of reps.

Spotting: The head stays neutral, neither looking upward or to the sides. The low back should not slouch downward (i.e., hyperextend).

Comments & Suggestions: The superman exercise occurs when the person is prone on the floor or bench and lifts the arms and legs upward at the same time. This modified version recruits more of the core musculature and is a good movement to enhance overall core stabilization. Those with weaker core muscles may have a smaller ROM. This is ok. Progress slowly as strength improves. For an added challenge, don't alternate limbs but rather perform all the reps on one side before moving to the other side (i.e., do 12 reps using the right arm/left leg; then do 12 reps using the left arm/right leg). Another name for this exercise is the *quadruped*.

BACK EXTENSION WITH STABILITY BALL

Primary Muscles Worked: Erector spinae.

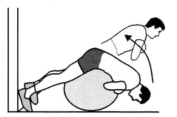

> **Quick Tip:** For added difficulty, don't anchor the feet to the wall.

Exercise Technique: Obtain a stability ball and lie face down (prone) on the ball with the belly button positioned near or at the top of the ball. The legs are hip to shoulder width apart and extended. There should be a slight bend in the knees. The feet can be pressed against a wall or ankles held by the trainer for added stability. The hands can be at the sides, crossed over the chest or stretched out in front, depending on the level of difficulty desired. Before the exercise begins, the lifter's trunk is flexed, which facilitates the upward concentric action. Concentric phase: Retract shoulder blades and slowly lift the upper body upward until it is approximately in line with the legs. Eccentric phase: Slowly lower to starting position. Repeat for the desired number of reps.

Spotting: Ensure retraction of shoulder blades throughout movement. The head should stay neutral. If stabilizing the lifter, hold at the ankles.

Comments & Suggestions: It is not necessary to hyperextend the back on this exercise. Also, for many people it's not necessary to use much added resistance (e.g., weight plates). Most people can be adequately challenged by lifting their body weight only. For most healthy people, several sets of 15-20 reps should be mastered before an external resistance is used (beginners may start with fewer reps than this). Back extensions may be inappropriate for people with some back injuries. Thus, if it hurts, try the modified superman described previously. For added difficulty, perform with the feet not anchored to wall or supported by a trainer. Difficulty increases (due to greater balance required) the closer the legs are to each other.

REVERSE BACK EXTENSION WITH STABILTY BALL

Primary Muscles Used: Erector spinae, gluteus maximus, hamstrings.

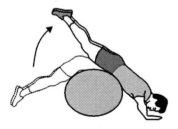

> **Quick Tip:** Begin with a small range of motion. Also try with knees bent.

Exercise Technique: Lie prone on a stability ball such that your head is lower than your hips. In this position the ball will be at about hip level. At this point the feet may either be slightly off the floor or just touching it. The legs should be extended (slight bend at knees), about hip width apart. The head is neutral and hands are on the floor facing forward, about shoulder width apart. The abs are tight. Concentric phase: Contract the glutes and slowly raise the legs upward until comfortable or until they are in line with body (approximately 45˚). Hold for a moment. Eccentric phase: Slowly lower legs to starting point. Repeat for the desired number of reps.

Spotting: The motion should be slow and controlled with no momentum. The legs should go no higher than the hips. Going further than this may cause the low back to hyperextend.

Comments & Suggestions: This exercise can also be performed with bent knees. It's important not to perform this exercise quickly. There should be no momentum. This exercise can also be performed on a bench if a stability ball is not available. Rise up slowly after completing because of possible temporary drops in blood pressure in some individuals.

CRUNCH ON STABILITY BALL

Primary muscles used: Rectus abdominis, internal and external obliques.

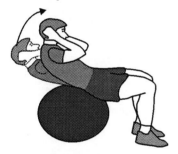

> **Quick Tip:** For added difficulty, try performing with one leg in the air.

Exercise Technique: Recline supine on a stability ball with feet about shoulder width apart and knees bent to about 90˚. When supine, the ball should rest somewhere between the low back to middle back range, depending on fitness level and difficulty desired. Concentric phase: Contract the abs (pull the belly button inward) and slowly curl the torso upward bringing the ribs closer to the hips. Eccentric phase: Slowly lower to starting point. Repeat for the desired number of reps.

Spotting: The upper torso should curl inward and become concave as it is lifted. Clasping the hands behind the neck may increase neck strain.

Comments & Suggestions: It's not necessary to curl all the way up until seated upright on the ball (although this can be a good teaching tool for learning how to stabilize on the ball prior to teaching the crunch). Just a slight movement is all that's needed to challenge the abs. If performed slowly, the abs should be sufficiently challenged after 12-20 reps. There are many ways to increase the difficulty of this exercise. For example, extending the arms over and behind the head or performing with one leg in the air increases difficulty. Placing the ball closer to the lower back area also increases difficulty. Some research suggests that greater abdominal recruitment occurs when the ball is placed closer to the low back region relative to performing crunches on the floor.[139] It's a myth that crunches selectively burn fat from the belly area.

REVERSE CRUNCH WITH STABILITY BALL

Primary Muscles Used: Rectus abdominis, internal and external obliques.

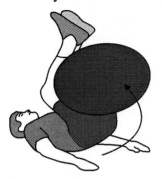

Quick Tip: For added difficulty, this can also be performed with different sized stability balls or with a medicine ball.

Exercise Technique: Obtain a stability ball and recline supine with bent legs over the ball about shoulder width apart. The back of the heels should press into the ball to aid in the lifting process. The arms should be at the sides, with hands facing down. Concentric phase: Contract the abdominals and slowly lift the ball into the air until comfortable or until the buttocks is slightly off the floor. Eccentric phase: Slowly lower the ball until it is almost touching the ground. Repeat for the desired number of reps.

Spotting: The head should be neutral. The low back should not come off the floor. If the ball touches the floor, it reduces tension on the abdominals.

Comments & Suggestions: Become proficient at performing the movement without a stability ball first. For added difficulty, lift the shoulders off the ground at the same time that the ball is lifted. It's very easy for the hip flexors to do all the work on this exercise especially when performed at a fast pace. Focus on working the abdominals.

OBLIQUE CRUNCH ON STABILITY BALL

Primary Muscles Used: Rectus abdominis, internal and external obliques, erector spinae.

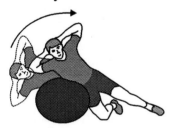

Quick Tip: Placing the feet against a wall makes this exercise easier.

Exercise Technique: Recline sideways on the stability ball as shown with the ball positioned at the midsection. The legs are extended with the inner leg behind the outer leg and flexed to aid with support. The outer leg should also be slightly bent. Concentric phase: Slowly lift the body upward, bringing the ribs closer to the hips. Hold for a second. Eccentric phase: Slowly lower body to the starting position. Repeat for the desired number of reps.

Spotting: The body should be centered equally on the ball. The head should be neutral.

Comments & Suggestions: Some recommend that the inner leg be extended with the outer leg behind it. Experiment to find which leg position works best for you. This is a challenging movement because less of the body is in contact with the ball. Bringing the legs closer increases the difficulty of this exercise. For more stability, perform with feet against a wall. This exercise does not selectively target fat loss from the sides of the abs or "love handles."

PRONE KNEE TUCK WITH STABILITY BALL

Primary Muscles Used: Abdominals (rectus abdominis, internal and external obliques), core musculature.

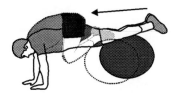

> **Quick Tip:** The exercise is harder when the ball is closer to the toes and even more difficult if performed with only one leg.

Exercise Technique: Obtain a stability ball and lie prone on it. Walk outward with your arms and hands so that you're in a push-up position. At this point the ball should be near the middle thighs (not pressing on the knees). Now slowly bend at the hip and knees, pulling the knees toward the chest. The ball is now moved closer to you. Then, slowly extend the legs and the ball moves back to its starting point. Repeat for the desired number of reps.

Spotting: The low back should not drop downward to the floor during this movement. The shoulder blades should not be squashed together. Rather, they should stay neutral. The head should be neutral also. The hands should be about shoulder width apart and oriented forward.

Comments & Suggestions: This exercise requires much upper body strength and balance. First, practice learning how to roll out and back on the ball before attempting this movement. Often considered an abdominal exercise, this movement uses many muscles including those of the chest, shoulders, upper and lower back and legs. The "core" which is also used, is sometimes thought of as consisting only of the abs and back muscles; however, the core really includes all the muscles of the trunk. The gluteals, for example, are included when we discuss the core.

PRONE SKIERS WITH STABILITY BALL

Primary Muscles Used: Abdominals, obliques, pectoralis major, deltoids, core musculature.

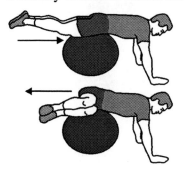

> **Quick Tip:** Performing with only one leg on the ball significantly increases the difficulty of this already challenging exercise.

Exercise Technique: While prone on a stability ball, roll forward until the ball is at the thighs. Arms are extended to the ground, under the shoulders and about shoulder width apart with a slight bend at the elbow. Hands are facing forward. The head is neutral. Contract the abs. Flex at the hips and bend at the knees, while moving the bent knees laterally to the side from the body until comfortable. Stop and return to the starting position. Perform the same action on the opposite side. Repeat.

Spotting: The low back should not bow downward (hyperextend). The head should stay neutral and the abs should be contracted.

Comments & Suggestions: This is a very challenging movement. Become proficient at the prone knee tuck before attempting. Start with a very small range of motion and increase slowly as strength and competency improves. One variation is to perform several reps on one side and then switch to the other side.

SUPINE LEG SCISSORS WITH STABILITY BALL

Primary Muscles Used: Abdominals (rectus abdominis, internal and external obliques).

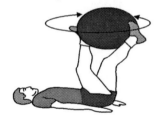

> **Quick Tip:** This exercise becomes harder as the extended legs get closer to the ground.

Exercise Technique: Recline supine with a stability ball clasped between the feet. The legs are in the air and extended upward (keep a slight bend at the knees) and slightly away from the body. The abs are contracted and the low back pressed into the ground. The arms are extended at the sides. Twirl the ball back and fourth between the feet by rotating the feet around the ball in a semi-circular pattern. At no time should the low back arch during the exercise.

Spotting: The low back should not arch up. Neither the upper body nor the head should come off the ground during the exercise.

Comments & Suggestions: While often considered an ab exercise, other muscles are also recruited (e.g., hip flexors). This exercise becomes harder as the extended legs get closer to the ground. A lower leg position also increases the stress on the low back. Discontinue if low back pain occurs.

Free Weights: Pros & Cons

Pro	Con
Inexpensive	Greater risk of injury
Adaptable to all sizes/shapes	Generally harder to use
Take up less space	Harder to isolate single muscle groups
Better activation of stabilizer & synergist muscles	Spotter generally needed for heavy lifts
Not limited to a fixed ROM	Requires greater coordination and skill
Less regular maintenance required	"Fear factor"

Machines: Pros & Cons

Pro	Con
Generally safer to use	Usually expensive
Generally easy to use	Generally uses a fixed ROM
Usually easier to isolate individual muscles	Generally heavy/bulky
Accommodating resistance	Some people may not fit in the machine
Easy to change resistances	More maintenance needed

Chapter 10

HOW HARD ARE PEOPLE EXERCISING?

This chapter will deal with some of the various ways that personal trainers use to determine exercise intensity. Both the clinical ways as well as the more-rubber-meets the road methods that fitness trainers use every day will be reviewed here.

VO2max Test

It is possible to determine how hard you are exercising by measuring how well your cells are using oxygen during exercise. This gives rise to what is called a VO2 test, where "V" stands for volume and "O2" is the chemical symbol for the oxygen that we breathe. Stated another way, VO2 is the volume of oxygen that is inhaled *minus* the volume of oxygen that is exhaled. Typically the test occurs while a person is exercising on a treadmill or a bicycle. An instrument, called a spirometer, is placed in the person's mouth and their nose is clamped off. The spirometer measures the volume of air that's breathed in and exhaled by the lungs. As you exercise, you will obviously breathe in more oxygen. Also, as the intensity of exercise is increased, you will use even more oxygen as you supply your body with the energy it needs to keep pace with the test. At some time during the test, however, a point is reached whereby the intensity of exercise becomes too difficult for your body to keep up. When this happens, you are exercising at your maximum ability and you have reached what is called *VO2max*. VO2max is the maximum volume of oxygen that can be taken into the body and used to make energy. Essentially, when you are at VO2max, *your pedal is to the metal* and you are working out as hard as you can. Studies show that an average VO2max for most people is around 30-40 ml O_2/kg BW/min, where *ml* stands for milliliters, *kg BW* is kilograms of body weight and *min* is minute. If you were speaking this to somebody, you would say "30 to 40 milliliters of oxygen per kilogram of body weight per minute." A kilogram is equal to 2.2 pounds. So essentially, this means that when most people are exercising at their maximum, every kilogram (2.2 pounds) of their body weight is consuming somewhere between 30 and 40 milliliters of oxygen per minute. An "athlete" or someone who works out at a high intensity on a regular basis is typically defined as someone who has a VO2max of above 50 ml O_2/kg BW/min.

Once VO2max is known, percentages of this can be calculated. People stay within this range when working out to foster the metabolic changes desired by the athlete. For generally healthy people, 60%-80% VO2max is usually recommended to support cardiovascular improvements.[25] It is important to note that VO2max is not just a measure of how well the lungs can take in oxygen. Rather, VO2max is the result of many body systems all working together for a common goal — energy production. VO2max involves the heart, lungs, red blood cells, arteries, veins, capillaries and even the size and number of mitochondria in the exercising muscles. VO2max is a concerted effort on the part of the body.

While typically measured in the lab, one field test that can estimate VO2max was developed by Dr. Kenneth Cooper, the founder of the modern aerobic exercise movement. In this equation, the person runs as far as possible in 12 minutes. This distance is converted to meters and the result is entered into this equation:

$$VO2max = \frac{D_{12} - 505}{45}$$

In this equation D_{12} is the distance (in meters) that a person runs in 12 minutes. Because of the complications associated with pushing an individual to their maximum limits, this may not be appropriate for all person's – especially if you conduct the test in an isolated area where help may not be available if something goes wrong. Field tests notwithstanding, clinically determining VO2max is the most accurate way we have to obtain a person's maximal aerobic capacity. The downside is that it's not often conducted in a typical health club setting because it requires expensive equipment. Because of this, fitness trainers typically estimate aerobic capacity based on a percentage of their estimated maximum heart rate, which we will discuss next.

Factors That Can Influence VO2max

Age	VO2max decreases as we age. Exercise can slow down this decline.
Altitude	Higher altitudes have less oxygen
Gender	Men tend to have a higher VO2max than women. This is not always the case and exercise can influence this.
Genetics	VO2max is greatly determined by our genes. Exercise might increase VO2max by about 20% in an untrained person.
Muscles	The muscle's ability to use oxygen
Heart	The heart's ability to pump blood
Lungs	The ability of the lungs to absorb oxygen
Blood	The ability of the blood to distribute oxygen to the body's tissues

Using Heart Rate

Because, in general, heart rate tends to increase when we exercise, we can use heart rate to estimate the difficulty of exercise. Let's now discuss the two most popular methods used to measure exercise intensity and then follow it up by reviewing other methods that fitness professionals should be familiar with.

Percent of Maximum Heart Rate

The foundation of this method is the equation, *220-Age*. By subtracting a person's age from the number 220 you can estimate the maximum number of times your heart will beat in one minute. For example, if you are 30 years old, 220 - 30 = 190bpm. Essentially this number means that "in theory" the heart of a 30-year-old person will be able to beat for no more than 190bpm if he/she is exercised to their maximum ability. You would never have anyone exercise at 100% of a person's maximum, so after this number is known, you calculate percentages of estimated maximal heart rate to arrive at what is sometimes called a target heart rate training zone or THR for short.

Normally we calculate two percentages and have people stay within that range. For example, you might calculate 60% and 80% of maximum heart rate. When the person gets fatigued, the pace is reduced until heart rate is closer to the lower level; when he/she feels better again, exercise intensity is increased to the end of the range.

Let's do an example so you can see how this method works. Suppose you were going to design a target heart rate zone of 60-75% for a healthy, 45-year-old female.

Step 1: 220 - 45 = 175bpm. (This is the person's estimated maximum heart rate)

Step 2: 175 x 0.60 = $\boxed{105\text{bpm}}$ and 175 x 0.75=$\boxed{131\text{bpm}}$

That's it! Your answer is 105bpm to 174bpm. Some may wonder how to multiply by a percent. All you have to do is move the decimal point two places to the left. Thus, in this example, 60% = 0.60 and 75% is 0.75.

It is important to remember that determination of maximal heart rate by the 220 minus Age equation is only an *estimation*. Research shows that actual maximal heart rate may be as much as 10-12 heart beats above or below what is calculated by the 220-Age equation.[1] Nevertheless, the equation is frequently used by fitness trainers because it is easy and convenient. Also, it is safer than exercising people to their maximum abilities and then calculating the THR. Many treadmills, bikes and other cardiovascular machines probably also use this equation when estimating heart rate. For example, treadmills etc. typically have programs called "fat burn" and "cardio." When you select one of these programs, you are prompted to enter your age. The machine the typically uses the 220-Age equation to determine exercise intensity. Usually the "fat burn zone" is supposed to be about 60% of maximum heart rate while the "cardiovascular zone" is at 80-85%. When using this equation with generally healthy individuals, it is usually stated that aerobic benefits occur at 70%-85% maximum heart rate.[1] Having said that, this range may be too much for some sedentary people to handle. This often causes confusion on the part of some new personal trainers who want a cut and dry answer to the question "what percentage range is best?" In reality, there is no perfect answer. As a personal trainer, you will look at the *whole person* when developing an effective and safe target heart rate range. You will look at their age, health issues, past experience with exercise, likes, dislikes, current/past injuries and goals and blend these together as best as you can to develop a target heart rate that's appropriate for that person.

Does a Baby's Heart Beat 220 Times a Minute?

People often wonder where the 220-Age formula came from. Since maximum HR is said to decline one beat per year from a supposed maximum of 220, does this mean that a baby's maximum rate is 220 beats per minute? Of course not! The 220-Age equation was invented because it seemed to best fit the data that scientists were seeing in their research. In other words, after looking at the numbers, it looked like maximum heart rate could be predicted by subtracting a person's age from 220. However, this research has been criticized by other investigators who highlight the lack of original research that specifically examined the validity of the 220-Age equation.[159] In other words, few studies exist which have actually tested whether the 220-Age equation really predicts with accuracy, the maximum heart rate. In fact, one of the criticisms against using this equation is that it might over- estimate or underestimate one's true maximum heart rate by as much 10-12 bpm according to some reports. Fitness professionals should be aware of this when they use this equation as their sole basis for prescribing an exercise target heart rate. In my opinion, the equation is used best when it is coupled with the other methods outlined in this chapter.

Karvonen Heart Rate Formula

The Karvonen heart rate formula can be thought of as an extension of percent of maximum heart rate formula just described. As such, this formula is usually considered to be a more accurate reflection of a person's aerobic stress during exercise. To use this formula you must first know a person's age and resting heart rate. When you know age and RHR, using the formula is pretty easy and has four steps. They are:

Karvonen Heart Rate Steps

Step 1:	220 - Age	
Step 2:	Subtract resting heart rate from step 1	
Step 3:	Multiply result of step 2 by percentages you wish to calculate	
Step 4:	Add resting heart rate to results of step 3	

The other name for the Karvonen formula is the *heart rate reserve* method. The heart rate reserve is simply the difference between maximal heart rate and resting heart rate. For example, if your maximum heart rate was 180bpm and your resting heart rate was 60bpm, your heart rate reserve is 180-60 = 120bpm. It is the heart rate reserve that is being calculated in step #2 of the Karvonen formula.

Some may wonder why we should calculate heart rate reserve when determining target heart rate ranges. Think of it this way. Simply taking percentages of maximal heart rate (220 – Age equation) does not take into consideration your resting heart rate. The heart rate reserve is the number of heart beats per minute that your heart can increase during exercise. In other words, it's your reserve heart beats. Think about it. Your heart rate does not increase from zero when you exercise! Rather, it increases from its resting rate (RHR) or some number above that. So, by subtracting your resting heart rate, you get a better picture of what your heart can do. Another interesting thing about the heart rate reserve is that as your fitness improves, your resting heart rate tends to decrease. This means that your reserve heart beats increase because the difference between maximal and resting heart rate grows larger. For example, if you were 30 years old and your RHR was 60bpm then your heart rate reserve is (220 - 30) – 60 = 130bpm. After six months of working out your RHR has dropped to 50bpm. This means that your heart rate reserve is now (220 - 30) – 50 = 140bpm. So, you gained an extra 10bpm that your heart can now increase during exercise!

Let's now illustrate how to use the Karvonen formula with an example. Suppose you wanted to use the formula to calculate a target heart rate range for a 45 year old healthy man who had a resting heart rate of 60bpm. You estimate that an intensity of 60% to 80% of his Karvonen max is enough to sufficiently tax his cardiovascular system safely.

Step 1: 220 – 45 = 175bpm

Step 2: 175 – 60 = 115bpm

Step 3: 115 X 60% = 69bpm   and   115 X 80% = 92bpm

Step 4: 69 + 60= $\boxed{129\text{bpm}}$ and   92 + 60 = $\boxed{152\text{bpm}}$

Your answer is 129bpm to 152bpm. You instruct the person to maintain a heart rate of between 129bpm and 152bpm, which corresponds to 60%-80% of his Karvonen HR max.

The Karvonen formula is usually said to be a more accurate reflection of a person's true aerobic ability. The reason for this is that it closely approximates a person's *percent of VO2max*, the "gold standard" of aerobic conditioning tests. In other words, if a person was working out at 60% of their Karvonen HR max, they would also be close to 60% of their VO2max. For most healthy person's, an intensity of 60%-80% of their Karvonen max is usually sufficient to obtain cardiovascular benefits when working out.[25]

It is important to remember that aerobic improvements can be achieved over a wide range of exercise intensities. Thus, the notion that everybody should work out at 60%-80% Karvonen max (or 60%-80% HR max) is not engraved in stone. People sometimes get hung up on these numbers and take them as gospel. In reality they are just guidelines for generally healthy people to strive toward. Having said that, is it possible for a generally healthy person to be unable to withstand this intensity for the often quoted 20-60 minutes a day? Of course! Personal training is "personal." As a fitness professional, you will likely run into people who are so deconditioned that a few minutes on a treadmill at a low intensity wipes them out! For some people, intermittent exercise may be best.

Exercise Intensities for Generally Healthy People

VO2max	60%-80%
Percent of Heart Rate Reserve (Karvonen Formula)	60%-80%
Percent of Maximum HR	70%-85%

When Not To Use Heart Rate

Once, while working at a health club, I encountered an older man who joined as a new member. My job at the time was to give new members a few tests to assess their general fitness. The health history form didn't present anything that seemed like a red flag to me and so I proceeded with the tests, one of which was a three minute step test used to gauge aerobic fitness. This test entailed that I take the resting heart rate before and after the person stepped up and down on an aerobic step for three minutes. Before the test I observed that the man's pulse was 60bpm. Immediately after the test, his pulse was still 60bpm! Since his pulse didn't change, I knew something was wrong. Looking over the health history questionnaire again, I noticed what I had not seen before. Stapled to the *back* of the form, was the note from his physician instructing me to not let his heart rate go above 100bpm! This man was on a medication called a *beta blocker*, a drug used to treat heart disease. One of the side effects of this medication is that it artificially slows down the resting heart rate. Because of my blunder I could have really hurt that man. Always remember that if you encounter a person who does not exercise and has a low resting heart rate, assume that they are on some medication that is slowing down the heart rate. In reality, one does not have to be "old" for this rule to apply; it's possible for someone in their 20's to be on beta blockers. When you encounter people who are on beta blockers or other medications that slow resting heart rate, you *cannot* use the Karvonen formula or the 200 – Age formula because they are based on heart rate. In this situation, the Borg Scale or Talk Test would be better options.

Other Ways To Measure How Hard Exercise Is

So, what do you do if you can't use heart rate to estimate exercise intensity? Fortunately, there are alternatives that you can use. This comes in handy when you are working with someone who may have a special need (e.g., high blood pressure).

The Talk Test

The talk test is one of the easiest ways to get an idea how hard someone is working out. In essence, if the person can talk while they are exercising, then they are deemed to not be exercising too hard. Some fitness books geared to the general public actually advocate this method to help people figure out for themselves if they are working out too hard or not. For example, it might be recommended that someone recite the Pledge of Allegiance while working out. If they can, they are doing ok.

It turns out that there is more to the talk test than simply saying the Pledge of Allegiance. Studies show that the point where speech first begins to get difficult, corresponds nicely with the *ventilatory threshold*.[26] Ventilation is the act of breathing in air and exhaling CO_2. As a rule of thumb, as exercise intensity increases, ventilation rate increases because you are breathing in and out faster to keep pace with your exercise. However, if the intensity of exercise is increased beyond a certain point (threshold), then your breathing increases dramatically. This is called the ventilatory threshold. If you were working with a client and wanted to use the Talk Test, just ask the person questions while they exercise aerobically. Sometimes people may start to mumble their answers. If this happens, ask them to speak up. Mumbling, or decreasing the pitch of their voice is their way of compensating and could be an indication that they are at or close to their ventilatory threshold. The ventilatory threshold usually starts to occur between 50%-80% VO2max (close to 50-80% Karvonen Max).[25] However, it's fitness level really determines when it kicks in, so relying on Karvonen may be inaccurate. Instead, just ask them questions and listen to their replies.

Are the Ventilatory and Lactate Thresholds the Same Thing?

Another term that usually gets mentioned when you start reading about ventilatory threshold is *lactate threshold* (lactate is a molecule formed during glycolysis when sugar is burned anaerobically). Another term for lactate threshold is *anaerobic threshold*. While the ventilatory threshold is the point where you start to breathe harder, the lactate threshold is the point during exercise when you begin to anaerobically produce large amounts of lactate. In other words, it's when the body starts to rely heavily on its anaerobic energy systems (primarily glycolysis) to meet its exercise energy needs. During this time, lactate production increases dramatically.

Borg Scale

The Borg Scale, also called ratings of perceived exertion (RPE scale) is a scale from 0-10 that people can use to indicate how difficult exercise feels to them. A rating of zero is "nothing at all" while a "10 is a maximum effort.

Rating	Meaning
0	Nothing at all
1	Very weak effort
2	Weak effort
3	Moderately strong or difficult effort
5	Strong or difficult effort
7	Very strong or difficult effort
10	Maximum effort

Where the numbers are not in perfect order (for example, between 5 and 7) it is understood that the number that is missing would be a level of intensity in-between. For example, in the table, level 6 is missing between level 5 and level 7. This indicates that level 6 is an intensity level between 5 and 7. The RPE scale is also an accepted method for gauging exercise intensity in people with high blood pressure/heart disease who use medications that lower RHR. One draw back to the RPE scale is that people must be familiar with what the numbers mean. In other words, asking someone how they feel on a zero to 10 scale may not produce an accurate result if the client has no idea what the numbers refer to.

The scale depicted here is actually a modified version of the original, 6-20 scale, where a rating of "6" was very light activity and "20" was maximum effort. One difference between the two versions is that the original 6-20 scale can also estimate exercise heart rate. For example, a rating of 6 is 6 x 10 or about 60 bpm. A rating of 20 is 20 x 10 or about 200 bpm. For the general population the 0-10 scale seems to be the more understandable of the two versions.

Metabolic Equivalents (METs)

If you take a close look at the displays on treadmills, ellipticals or other pieces of cardiovascular equipment, there is a chance you have noticed METs but not given much thought to it. METs, however, provides a very useful tool that you can use to monitor how difficult exercise is. METs, or *metabolic equivalents,* are basically a comparison between exercise metabolic rate and resting (or sleeping) metabolic rate. More specifically, we know that all humans burn (use) approximately 3.5 milliliters of oxygen per kilogram of their body weight per minute. This is 1 MET and is usually abbreviated as 3.5 ml O_2/kg BW/ min. This is spoken as "3.5 milliliters of oxygen per kilogram of bodyweight per minute." A kilogram is equal to 2.2 pounds. So, if we could remove a 2.2 pound chunk from your thigh, etc., and measure the amount of oxygen it is using when you are resting, we would find that it is burning about 3.5 millimeters of oxygen per minute. If you were thinking that this sounds a lot like VO2, you are correct because METs and VO2 are very similar. Essentially, they are the same thing, just spoken in different "languages." In fact, 1 MET is actually your resting VO2![29]

Other Names for 1 MET

1 MET is also:

- Resting VO2
- Basal metabolic rate (BMR)
- Amount of calories burned at rest

Since METs and VO2 are basically the same thing and since 1 MET is 3.5 ml O2/kg BW/ min, we can use this number to convert from METs to VO2 and back again. For example, suppose you were working out on a treadmill and the readout said you were at 5 METs. What is your VO2?

If 1 MET = 3.5 ml/kg BW/ min.

Then 5 METs = 5 X 3.5 = $\boxed{17.5 \text{ ml/kg BW/ min}}$

Essentially, you just multiplied the MET number by 3.5 to get the corresponding VO2. This answer of 17.5 ml O2/kg BW/min is based on a kilogram (2.2 lb) basis. In other words, each kilogram (2.2 pounds) of the person's body weight is consuming 17.5 ml of oxygen per minute. If you wanted to obtain the actual VO2 at which the person was working, you would multiply the VO2 by the person's weight. For example, if the person weighed 180 pounds (82 kg) you would multiply 17.5 X 82 kg = 1435 milliliters of oxygen per minute.

METs and Metabolism

Remember that while 1 MET equals 3.5 ml O2/kg BW/ min, this is on a *per kilogram basis*. People of different weights will consume different total amounts of oxygen at rest. Take two people, for example. One weighs 100 kg and the other 50 kg. Both use about 3.5 ml/kg BW/ min but the total oxygen they use at rest is 100 x 3.5 = 350 ml O2 & 50 kg X 3.5 =175 ml O2. Looking at this from another angle, since oxygen consumption is related to metabolism, heavier people will generally have *higher* metabolic rates than thinner people. This is food for thought when dealing with overweight clients who feel their metabolism is low or sluggish.

Now, suppose you know the VO2 but wanted to know the MET level at which the person was working. In this instance you just divide the VO2 by 3.5. In the example above, the VO2 is 17.5 ml O2/kg BW/ min. To determine METs at this workload, divide 17.5 by 5 = 5 METs.

Let's say you don't care about converting METs to VO2. You can still use METs to determine how hard exercise feels. Remember that 1 MET also represents your lowest metabolic rate, BMR (this is where *metabolic* comes from in metabolic equivalents). BMR can be thought of as the calories you are burning when you're sleeping. So, if you are working out at 2 METs, that means you're burning calories twice has fast as when you're sleeping. If the treadmill says you're working out at 10 METs, you're burning calories 10 times faster than sleeping! In general, moderate activity is defined as 3-6 METs while vigorous activity is defined as more than 6 METs.[35] Keep in mind that the age, physical limitations and fitness level of a person also factor in to what is easy or difficult. For example, it may be easy for a 30-year-old woman to walk to the neighborhood store but very difficult for someone who is 80 or who has physical disabilities. This makes quantifying different activities according to METs difficult for all people. When in doubt, it's wise to use METs with the RPE scale and/or the Talk Test to get a better picture of the difficulty of exercise.

It's important for fitness professionals have a working understanding of METs because they are used clinically to gauge exercise intensity. It's possible that one day you will encounter a person carrying a note from a physician that stipulates that the patient not exercise more than a certain MET level. If you have access to treadmills or bikes that measure METs, this person can be easily accommodated.

In healthy and unhealthy people, evidence suggests that the risk of dying from all causes decreases as cardiovascular fitness improves.[123,124,125] In fact, research finds that on average, each 1 MET increase in exercise capacity might improve survival by 12% in healthy and non-healthy men.[123] In women, these results appear to be even greater with every increase of 1 MET improving survival by 17%[125]. But, how much exercise does it take to do this? The Surgeon General recommends that everyone engage in moderate physical activity most days of the week (i.e., at least 4 days), if not every day. Other research suggests that burning 2000 calories per week can significantly improve health. With respect to METs, the following equations can be used to estimate the "target MET level" men and women should strive for when working out.[124]

Determining Target MET Level

Gender	Equation
Men	14.7 - (0.11 x your age)
Women	14.7 - (0.13 x your age)

For example, a healthy 40 year old woman should strive to exercise aerobically at an intensity of: 14.7 - (0.13 X 40) = 14.7- 5.2 = 9.5METs. If achieving this level is not possible, do to health reasons, another goal would be to reach at least 85% of the value calculated by these equations. Some research finds double the rates of death in women whose fitness is less than 85% of that predicted by the female equation.[124] Regardless of the numbers, much evidence suggests that improved physical fitness can help reduce the risk of death in both men and women. METs can be a powerful tool to help educate people to stay healthy. If health reasons prevent the achievement of the target MET level, remember that physical activity in general will improve health. In other words, doing anything is better than doing nothing at all.

Chapter 11

FITNESS TESTING

Fitness testing is what fitness professionals do to get an idea of a person's overall fitness level. This is usually determined soon after the association between client and trainer begins. There is, of course, no single perfect measure of a person's overall fitness. This is why various aspects of fitness are usually determined. The most common aspects of fitness are as follows:

1. **Muscular strength:** The ability of a muscle to exert force.
2. **Muscular endurance:** The ability of a muscle to contract repeatedly over time.
3. **Cardiovascular endurance:** The ability of the heart, lungs and blood vessels to deliver oxygen and nutrients to the exercising muscles and remove waste products.
4. **Flexibility:** The range of motion of a joint.
5. **Body composition:** The amount of muscle and fat present on the body.

Some also add *balance* to this list, because through aging, disuse and various medical conditions, balance detriments may also be observed. For example, many older adults will have poor balance. These values, once known, can be compared to other people of the same age and gender to determine where a person ranks. Each of the parameters of fitness can be tested. Some of the more common tests for each aspect of fitness are described below: Keep in mind that these are not the only tests available. You may have used or heard about other tests that are not measured here.

Muscular Strength Tests

10RM Test

One way to measure muscular strength is to determine the most weight that a person can lift for a certain number of times. This is sometimes referred to as an *RM test*. The letters RM stand for Repetition Maximum and represent the most weight that a person can lift for a specific number of repetitions with good lifting technique. For example, a weight that is equal to a person's 10 RM is a weight that can only be lifted 10 times with good lifting form. Usually a test for upper body and lower body strength is determined. Classic examples include the bench press for upper body strength and leg press for lower body strength. To determine the upper and lower body 10RM for someone, follow these steps:

1. Warm up. After becoming familiar with the equipment, warm up for 5 to 10 minutes with a low-intensity aerobic activity. In addition, one may also incorporate a more activity-specific warm-up like performing a set of low intensity bench presses or leg presses to warm up the muscles even more.
2. Choose a weight that you feel the client can lift *only* 10 times. Be conservative when choosing and do not overestimate what you think the person can lift. If the person can lift more than 10 repetitions, rest 2-5 minutes and repeat the test with a heavier weight. For the bench press, increase the weight by 5-10 pounds. For the leg press, increase 10-

30 pounds. Continue the test until a load that can only be lifted 10 times with good lifting form is determined. Ideally, the 1RM should be found in 3 to 5 trials.[1]

Some may choose to determine 1RM or the most weight that a person can lift only one time with good lifting technique. This, according to the ACSM, is the "gold standard" of strength testing.[1] Because it entails lifting a considerable about of weight, some feel it's controversial because of thoughts that it might carry an increased risk of injury. While this is debatable, it may not be appropriate for beginners or those with medical issues. Those who determine 1RM directly should remember that 1RM testing is also not appropriate for smaller muscle groups. For example, attempting a 1RM lift with a biceps curl or triceps extension may damage these joints. It is for this reason that 1RM is usually only recommended for the large upper and lower body muscles. Any large muscle group exercise that places a person in a risky position (e.g., unsupported bent over row) is generally not appropriate for 1RM testing.

The fact that different people of the same age and gender can usually lift different amounts of weight is the reason why tables listing various 1RM weights are impractical. However, when maximum weight pushed (1RM) is divided by a person's body weight, it is possible to generate a table that can rank a person's 1RM for various ages. The following are tables for the bench press and leg press—the most often used measures of upper and lower body strength.

1RM Bench Press Strength Values for Men (1RM /Bodyweight)[1,5]

Ranking	20-29	30-39	40-49	50-59	>60
90	1.48	1.24	1.10	0.97	0.89
80	1.32	1.12	1.00	0.90	0.82
70	1.22	1.04	0.93	0.84	0.77
60	1.14	0.98	0.88	0.79	0.72
50	1.06	0.93	0.84	0.75	0.68
40	0.99	0.88	0.80	0.71	0.66
30	0.93	0.83	0.76	0.68	0.63
20	0.88	0.78	0.72	0.63	0.57
10	0.80	0.71	0.65	0.57	0.53

Percentile Ranking: 90 = well above average; 70=above average; 50 = average; 30 = below average; 10=well below average

1 RM Bench Press Strength Values for Women (1RM/Bodyweight)[1,5]

Ranking	20-29	30-39	40-49	50-59	>60
90	0.54	0.49	0.46	0.40	0.41
80	0.49	0.45	0.40	0.37	0.38
70	0.42	0.42	0.38	0.35	0.36
60	0.41	0.41	0.37	0.33	0.32
50	0.40	0.38	0.34	0.31	0.30
40	0.37	0.37	0.32	0.28	0.29
30	0.35	0.34	0.30	0.26	0.28
20	0.33	0.32	0.27	0.23	0.26
10	0.30	0.27	0.23	0.19	0.25

Percentile Ranking: 90 = well above average; 70=above average; 50 = average; 30 = below average; 10=well below average

1 RM Leg Press Strength Values for Men (1RM /Bodyweight)[1,5]

Ranking	20-29	30-39	40-49	50-59	>60
90	2.27	2.07	1.92	1.80	1.73
80	2.13	1.93	1.82	1.71	1.62
70	2.05	1.85	1.74	1.64	1.56
60	1.97	1.77	1.68	1.58	1.49
50	1.91	1.71	1.62	1.52	1.43
40	1.83	1.65	1.57	1.46	1.38
30	1.74	1.59	1.51	1.69	1.30
20	1.63	1.52	1.44	1.32	1.25
10	1.51	1.43	1.35	1.22	1.16

Percentile Ranking: 90 = well above average; 70=above average; 50 = average; 30 = below average; 10=well below average

1 RM Leg Press Strength Values for Women (1RM /Bodyweight)[5]

Ranking	20-29	30-39	40-49	50-59	>60
90	2.05	1.73	1.63	1.51	1.40
80	1.66	1.50	1.46	1.30	1.25
70	1.42	1.47	1.35	1.24	1.18
60	1.36	1.32	1.26	1.18	1.15
50	1.32	1.26	1.19	1.09	1.08
40	1.25	1.21	1.12	1.03	1.04
30	1.23	1.16	1.06	0.95	0.98
20	1.13	1.09	0.94	0.86	0.94
10	1.02	0.94	0.76	0.75	0.84

Percentile Ranking: 90 = well above average; 70=above average; 50 = average; 30 = below average; 10=well below average

For example, suppose a 30-year-old man who weighed 185 lbs had a 1RM of 350 lbs on the leg press. Doing the math, this equals 350 ÷ 185 =1.89. According to this number, the person is in the 70th percentile for his age and gender for the leg press.

For those who do not want to directly determine 1RM, it is possible to estimate this value with the use of lighter loads and equations. One such equation used to estimate 1RM is the following:[6]

$$1RM = (number\ of\ reps\ /\ 30) + 1) \times weight\ lifted$$

For example. Suppose a person could lift 150 pounds 10 times. According to the equation, 1RM = ((10 reps / 30) +1) X 150 pounds= 200 pounds. So, her 1RM = 200 lbs.

It should be stressed that the number arrived at by this equation (and other equations not mentioned) is only an estimation and may not completely reflect a person's true 1 RM. Because of this, some choose to determine 1RM directly. Before doing so, however people should weigh the risks and benefits of directly determining 1RM before attempting.

Grip Strength Test

This test requires the use of a device called a dynamometer. Usually the dynamometer is held in the hand and squeezed as hard as possible. This test measures isometric hand strength, which is taken as an indicator of overall body strength. While relatively easy to do, the grip strength test may not accurately reflect real life strength. In other words, weak grip strength may not correspond to weak overall strength.

Muscular Endurance Tests

Push-Up Test

In this test, we record the maximum number of good-form push-ups that can be performed. The male client assumes a normal push-up stance while for some females, a bent-knee modified version may be used. It is important to remember that for some individuals, like seniors or those with weak upper body strength, push-ups are very difficult to perform. Because of this, the push-up test may end up being a measure of *muscle strength* and not muscle endurance. In addition, the push-up test may be inappropriate for people who have shoulder or low back problems.

Push-Up Test Percentile Rankings for Men[1]

Ranking	20-29	30-39	40-49	50-59	60-69
90	41	32	25	24	24
80	34	27	21	17	16
70	30	24	19	14	11
60	27	21	16	11	10
50	24	19	13	10	9
40	21	16	12	9	7
30	18	14	10	7	6
20	16	11	8	5	4
10	11	8	5	4	2

Percentile Ranking: 90 = well above average; 70=above average; 50 = average; 30 = below average; 10=well below average

Push-Up Test Percentile Rankings for Women[1]

Ranking	20-29	30-39	40-49	50-59	60-69	>70
90	31	27	25	19	18	24
80	27	22	21	17	15	17
70	21	20	17	13	13	11
60	19	17	16	12	11	9
50	18	16	14	11	9	7
40	14	13	11	9	6	2
30	13	10	10	6	4	0
20	10	7	8	3	0	0
10	6	1	4	0	0	0

Percentile Ranking: 90 = well above average; 70=above average; 50 = average; 30 = below average; 10=well below average

146

Bench Press Test

This test, popularized by the YMCA (hence its alternate name, YMCA Bench Press Test) is similar to the timed push-up test described previously. Men use an 80-pound barbell and women use a 35-pound barbell.[4] This test measures the number of repetitions a barbell can be lifted at a cadence of 30 lifts per minute while reclined on a flat bench.[4] The speed of the lift is set with the use of a metronome. The test is terminated when the person cannot keep up with the metronome cadence.

YMCA Bench Press Percentile Rankings by Age[3,5]

Age	18-25		26-35		36-45		46-55		56-65		Over 65	
Ranking	M	F	M	F	M	F	M	F	M	F	M	F
90	44	42	41	40	36	33	28	29	24	24	20	18
80	37	34	33	32	29	28	22	22	20	20	14	14
70	33	28	29	28	25	24	20	18	14	14	10	10
60	29	25	26	24	22	21	16	14	12	12	10	8
50	26	21	22	21	20	17	13	12	10	9	8	6
40	22	18	20	17	17	14	11	9	8	6	6	4
30	20	16	17	14	14	12	9	7	5	5	4	3
20	16	12	13	12	10	8	6	5	3	3	2	1
10	10	6	9	6	6	4	2	1	1	1	1	0

Percentile Ranking: 90 = well above average; 70=above average; 50 = average; 30 = below average; 10=well below average

Another way to gauge muscle endurance is to have the person complete a series of 7 exercises for upper and lower body. This method has the advantage of determining muscle endurance over a wide range of muscle groups and, as such, may be a better predictor of total body muscle endurance. For each exercise, the person lifts a percentage of his/her body weight.[3] The maximum goal for each exercise should be 15 repetitions. Thus, a maximum score for all seven exercises is 7 X 15 = 105 total repetitions lifted. The following table lists the exercises to use in this battery of tests, as well as the corresponding percentage of body weight that each station should include.

Muscle Endurance Battery of Exercises[3]

Percent of body weight to be lifted

Exercise	Men	Women	Reps performed (max=15)
Bench press	0.66	0.50	
Lat pull down	0.66	0.50	
Leg extension	0.50	0.50	
Leg curl	0.33	0.33	
Triceps extension	0.33	0.33	
Biceps curl	0.33	0.25	
Bent-knee sit-up	Not applicable	Not applicable	
		Total # of Reps (max=105)	Total =

For example, using the values from the table, if a man weighed 150 lbs and was performing a bench press, he would lift 150 lbs X 0.66 = 99 pounds. If he were performing the leg curl, he would lift 150 X 0.33 = 49.5 pounds. He would try to complete a maximum of 15 repetitions on each exercise test. No percent of body weight is associated with sit-ups. The maximum number of reps that should be attempted to be performed for all tests combined is 105. Make sure all repetitions are with good lifting technique to avoid overstraining or injury. Use the following categories when scoring this test[3]:

Total Reps Completed		Meaning
91-105 repetitions	=	Excellent
77-90 repetitions	=	Very good
63-76 repetitions	=	Good
49-62 repetitions	=	Fair
35-48 repetitions	=	Poor
Less than 35 repetitions	=	Very poor

Timed Sit-Up Test

This test measures the muscle endurance of the hip flexors and abdominals. In this test, the person is supine on a padded mat with arms crossed over the chest, touching the shoulders, and knees bent in the usual sit-up position. When the test begins, the person curls up until his/her torso is perpendicular with the floor (i.e., straight up). Immediately thereafter, the person lowers his/her torso until their shoulder blades are on the mat. The person repeats this for as many times as possible for one minute. Those who cannot complete one minute of continuous abdominal contractions are allowed to rest during the test. However, resting will not affect the time limit of the test. In other words, the test will be over in one minute whether the person rests or not. The sit-up test may not be appropriate for individuals who have low back or neck issues, osteoporosis, large abdominal girths or in those who cannot get up from the floor after the test is over.

Sit-Up Test (YMCA test) Percentile Rank by Age/Gender[5]

Age	18-25		26-35		36-45		46-55		56-65		Over 65	
Ranking	M	F	M	F	M	F	M	F	M	F	M	F
90	77	68	62	54	60	54	61	48	56	44	50	34
80	66	61	56	46	52	44	53	40	49	38	40	32
70	57	57	52	41	45	38	51	16	46	32	35	29
60	52	51	44	37	43	35	44	33	41	27	31	26
50	46	44	38	34	36	31	39	31	36	24	27	22
40	41	38	36	32	32	28	33	28	32	22	24	20
30	37	34	33	28	29	23	29	25	28	18	22	16
20	33	32	30	24	25	20	24	21	24	12	19	16
10	27	25	21	20	21	16	16	13	20	8	12	11

Percentile Ranking: 90 = well above average; 70=above average; 50 = average; 30 = below average; 10=well below average9

Curl-Up Test

Because sit-ups involve the hip flexor muscles, some favor a modified version that utilizes crunches or partial abdominal curls. This test has two variations. One form of the test has the person complete as many crunches as possible in one minute. In this respect the test is very similar to the timed sit up test described previously. The other version requires the use of a metronome set to 40 beats per minute (which should allow 20-curl ups per minute). The person, supine on a mat with arms at sides, curls his/her torso up to the point that the shoulder blades are off the floor and then returns to the starting point, while keeping pace with the metronome. This continues for as many times as can be completed up to a maximum of 75 repetitions. Like the sit-up test, the curl-up test may not be appropriate for those with osteoporosis, large midsections, older individuals or those who cannot get up from the floor.

Partial Curl-Up Percentile Rankings[1]

Age	20 - 29		30 - 39		40 - 49		50 - 59		60 - 69	
Ranking	M	F	M	F	M	F	M	F	M	F
90	75	70	75	55	75	50	74	48	53	50
80	56	45	69	43	75	42	60	30	33	30
70	41	37	46	34	67	33	45	23	26	24
60	31	32	36	28	51	28	35	16	19	19
50	27	27	31	21	39	25	27	9	16	13
40	24	21	26	15	31	20	23	2	9	9
30	20	17	19	12	26	14	19	0	6	3
20	13	12	13	0	21	5	13	0	0	0
10	4	5	0	0	13	0	0	0	0	0

Percentile Ranking: 90= well above average; 70=above average; 50= average; 30= below average; 10=well below average

Cardiovascular Endurance Tests

Cardiovascular endurance (CV endurance) refers to the ability of the heart, lungs and blood vessels to deliver adequate oxygen and nutrients to the exercising muscles while at the same time removing waste products that build up and hinder exercise performance. Looking at the big picture, two different paths can be taken to determine CV Fitness: maximal exercise testing and submaximal exercise testing. Maximal exercise testing has a higher degree of accuracy; but, it also carries a greater risk of injury (e.g., heart attack). Because of the risks involved, maximal exercise testing should only be performed in the presence of a physician. Submaximal exercise testing is how fitness professionals usually determine CV endurance. Here, people are exercised at lower intensities. The information obtained from the test can then be entered into an equation to estimate CV fitness. Cardiovascular endurance is different than muscular endurance, described previously. Because of this, different tests are needed to gauge cardiovascular endurance. The following are some of the more common submaximal CV endurance tests used by fitness professionals.

Rockport Walking Test

This test involves having a person walk one mile as fast as possible. The pulse is then taken for one minute immediately after exercise and entered into an equation to determine CV Fitness. Because only fast walking is required, this test would be expected to have a lower risk of injury than tests that involve running. The equation used to determine CV Fitness for the Rockport walking test is[3]:

132.853 - (0.0769 × Weight) - (0.3877 × Age) + (6.315 × Gender) - (3.2649 × Time) - (0.1565 × Heart rate)

For gender, use 1 for males and 0 for females.

When computing the answer, remember that various computer programs are available which can do the math for you. For those who do not have access to these programs, many websites can also help. If you use the internet, remember to double check the answer on several other websites to make sure you are getting a valid answer.

The Rockport walking test has been shown to be effective in men and women age 20-69.[3] Fitness trainers should keep in mind that what is "fast walking" for one person may be very different than for another person. Thus, a 69-year-old man will probably walk slower than a 25-year-old female.

The 1.5-Mile Run Test

In this test, the person is instructed to cover a distance of 1.5 miles as quickly as possible. Walking is allowed during the test for those who cannot run the complete distance, although the person should be instructed to complete the distance as fast as he/she can. Stretching and warm-up occur prior to the test. From this test, the VO2max of the individual can be estimated from the equation[3]:

VO2max = 88.02 – (0.1656 x body weight in kilograms) – (2.76 x time) + (3.716 x gender)

With respect to *gender* in the equation, enter either 1 for men or 0 for women. An average VO2max for many adults will usually be around 30 - 40 ml 0_2/ kg BW / min, while fit people would be above 50 ml 0_2/ kg BW / min.

Other points about this equation to remember:

1. The person's weight is in kilograms. To convert to Kg, divide body weight (in lbs) by 2.2

2. The time it took to cover the 1.5 miles should be in minutes. If the distance was not covered in an exact minute (e.g., 10 minutes exactly), convert the seconds into minutes by dividing the seconds by 60. For example, if it took a person 10 minutes and 20 seconds to complete the 1.5 miles, divide the 20 seconds by 60 = 0.33. Thus, the person completed the distance in 10.33 minutes.

1.5-Mile Run Example

Suppose you were testing a 21-year-old female who weighs 120 lbs. She completed the 1.5-mile run in 9 minutes, 10 seconds. Use the 1.5-mile run equation to estimate her VO2max.

Step 1. Convert her weight to kg. 120 lbs ÷ 2.2 = 55 kg
Step 2. Convert 9 min 10 seconds to all minutes. 10 ÷ 60 =0.17. Thus, she ran the 1.5-mile distance in 9.17 minutes.
Step 3. She is female, so the conversion factor for the equation is 0.

Let's break the equation down into 3 parts to make it easier:

Part 1. $88.02 - (0.1656 \times 55)$ $88.02 - (9.1) = 78.9$

Part 2. $78.9 - (2.76 \times 9.17) = 78.9 - (25.3) = 53.6$

Part 3. $53.6 + (3.716 \times 0) = 53.6 + 0 = \boxed{53.6}$

Answer: Her VO2max is about 53.6 ml O2 / kg BW / min.

The 1.5-mile run is a relatively good test of cardiovascular (aerobic) endurance; but, keep in mind that there is not total agreement that the ability to run for certain distances equals an accurate indicator of VO2max.[2] The calculation of VO2max would be less precise in those who cannot run the complete distance or in those who take rest breaks during the test. The test may also not be appropriate in those who have arthritis or other bone/joint disorders, balance problems or in the elderly. Another issue to consider with this test is that it typically is performed outside where help may not be readily available if an accident occurs.

12-Minute Walk/Run

This test is similar to the 1.5-mile run but is a little less demanding because walking is allowed. Usually a flat surface like a walking track is used, although a variation of this test could incorporate a treadmill. If a walking track is used, break the track into different sections (e.g., every 10th of a mile) to better determine the distance covered. In this test, the person is instructed to cover as much distance as they can in 12 minutes. This can be accomplished either by walking, running or some combination of both. Stretching before the test might help reduce injury. The distance covered can be used to estimate VO2max. The equation used to estimate VO2max is:

$$VO2max = (0.0268 \times distance\ covered) - 11.3$$

The distance in this equation is in meters. Thus, if you are working with miles you will have to first convert miles to meters before using this equation. One mile equals about 1,600 meters. So, if the person ran/walked 2.5 miles in twelve minutes, this equals: $(2 \times 1600) + (0.5 \times 1600) = 3200 + 800 = 4000$ meters.

Treadmill Fit Test

Some treadmills and stationary bikes have a built-in 5-minute "Fit Test" that can be used to estimate CV fitness. This test requires no math on the part of the fitness professional – the fit test does all the work! While the fit test cannot diagnose any cardiovascular problems, it does give estimates of VO2max and also indicates how the person compares to others of similar age and gender (e.g., excellent, poor, fair, good).

Flexibility Tests

Flexibility is defined as the ability of a joint to move through a full range of motion (ROM). A joint is defined as any where two bones meet (e.g., knee joint or elbow joint). Different joints will have different degrees of ROM. For example, the shoulder joint has the greatest ROM in the body. This also comes at the cost of being one of the most easily injured joints in the body as well. Flexibility depends on a number of issues, including, but limited to, the inflexibility or tightness of ligaments or tendons, age (flexibility tends to decrease as we age), activity level (lack of physical activity correlates with being inflexible), posture (poor posture may lead to inflexible joints) and even the amount of body fat a person has. Some research even suggests that women may have greater flexibility in some joints than men.[3] Various methods exist to test flexibility. Fitness professionals should remember that no single test can determine the flexibility of all the joints in the body simultaneously.

Sit and Reach Test

This is a popular test of hamstring and low back flexibility. Following a brief warm-up of simple stretches, the person sits on the floor with legs extended but not locked. A yardstick can be placed on the floor between the person's legs. A piece of tape is placed on the floor at the 15-inch mark on the yard stick. The person is instructed to slowly reach forward, with arms stretched (hands over each other) as far as possible, hold for a moment and relax. Make sure that during the test the knees do not bend and that the person doesn't compensate by reaching further with one hand. Record the distance. Repeat this test three times. The furthest point reached is recorded as their low back and hamstring flexibility.

Some may choose to use a *sit and reach box* to perform this test. When using the sit-and-reach box, the person removes their shoes and sits on the floor with feet against the base of the box and legs straight, about shoulder-width apart. The starting position when using a sit-and-reach box is 26 centimeters. This is called the "zero point." After 3 practice tests, extend the arms and, with hands over each other and palms down, reach forward slowly as far as comfortable. Record the distance. Repeat this test 3 times and record the best distance.

Body Composition Tests

Being overweight is defined as having an excess of body weight for one's height and age. The term *obese* is reserved for those who have a body mass index (BMI) of 30 kg/m^2 or more.[1] "Morbid obesity" is defined as being over 100 lbs overweight or having a BMI of 35-40 or more.[160] Body composition generally refers to the amount of muscle and fat a person has. Body fat can be further broken down into *essential fat* (about 3% in men and 15% in women) and *storage fat* which is everything other than storage fat. It is sometimes necessary to measure body composition to get a better idea of an individual's general health and disease risk classification.

Average Body Fat Percentages[2]

	Men	Women
Average	12%-15%	22%-25%
Obese	Grater than 25	Greater than 30%

Health Risks Associated with Being Overweight[7]*

Premature death from all causes	Type II diabetes	Breast cancer	Pregnancy-related complications
Heart disease	Colon cancer	Endometrial cancer	Gestational diabetes
High blood pressure	Gall bladder cancer	Sleep apnea	Increased surgical risks
Elevated triglycerides	Prostate cancer	Asthma	Irregular menstrual cycles
Decreased HDL	Kidney cancer	Arthritis	Incontinence

*Partial list

Several common measures are available to assess body composition. While some tests are more accurate than others, all have their limitations and drawbacks. Thus, there is no "perfect" test for everybody. The trick is to choose a test that is reasonably accurate and is easy to duplicate over time. The following are the more common types of body composition tests that fitness trainers should be aware of.

Body Weight Scales

Many individuals use household scales to estimate their weight. However, the scale only provides one raw number (total body weight). Scales can, however, be a valuable tool to keep track of body weight and help track weight loss efforts. On the downside, scales do not distinguish between fat mass and muscle mass. For example, the scale may not show the full picture in a person who is gaining muscle while losing fat.

Body Typing

Body typing attempts to classify people into one of three types: *ectomorph, mesomorph* or *endomorph*. The ectomorph is said to be thin and have a hard time gaining weight. Endomorphs are said to have a hard time losing weight. Mesomorphs are defined as having a muscular build and narrow waist. Problems with this type of analysis include the fact that it doesn't consider percent body fat and not everybody fits into these three classifications. Also, in theory, classifying according to body types may provide people with a *crutch* that prevents attainment of goals.

Height–Weight Tables

Height-weight tables determine body composition based on gender and the size of one's frame. Like scales, height-weight tables do not assess the amount of body fat a person has. Rather, they compare people to an "average" person. Problems abound when using only these tables for body composition analysis. For example, many professional athletes are considered overweight when assessed with height-weight tables.[8] Because of error and because other, better methods exist, the fitness professional should not rely solely on height-weight tables to determine body composition.

Body Mass Index

The body mass index (BMI) is very popular in some circles and is a comparison of how tall a person is, relative to how much they weigh. It is easy to determine and only requires a scale and tape measure. The BMI is usually calculated from the equation:

$$BMI = weight\ (in\ kilograms) \div height\ (in\ meters^2)$$

That is, one calculates BMI as the weight of a person (in kilograms) divided by the person's height (in meters squared). This is written in the form kg/m^2. For example, if a person weighed 200 lbs. and was six feet tall, his BMI would be calculated the following way:

1. Convert pounds to kilograms. Since there are 2.2 lbs in a kilogram, 200 lb. ÷ 2.2 = 91 kg.

2. Convert the person's height to meters squared (m^2). Since the person is six feet tall and since there are 3.28 feet in a meter, the person is 1.8 meters tall (6 ÷ 3.28). Now square this amount (that is, 1.8 meters X 1.8 meters) to get 3.24m^2.

3. The person's BMI is 91 kg / 3.24m^2 = $\boxed{28.0 \text{ kg/m}^2}$

Another BMI equation that does not rely on the metric system is:

$$BMI = 703 \text{ (weight in pounds} \div \text{height}^2 \text{ in inches)}$$

BMI is useful as a quick test of a person's disease risk because many obesity-related health problems tend to increase as BMI increases over 25 kg/m^2 for most people.[2] For example, on average a person with a BMI of 18-25 runs up about $4000 annually in healthcare costs while in those whose BMI is over 40, this amount almost doubles to about $8000 annually.[161] According to current guidelines, a BMI of 25-29 kg/m^2 is classified as "overweight" and a BMI of over 30 kg/m^2 is considered "obese." While BMI offers a quick and relatively easy way to assess a person's' body composition, it does have its limitations. For example, many professional athletes are classified as "obese" via BMI. This is because BMI does not differentiate between muscle and fat. Two people can be the same height and weight and thus have the same BMI, yet one person may have 10% body fat while another may have 35%. In addition, there is a ± 5% error when determining body fatness from BMI.[1,2] While a valuable tool, BMI alone may not give the full picture of a person's health.

Body Mass Index

BMI	Meaning
18.5-24.9	Healthy weight
25-29.9	Overweight
> 30	Obese
30-34.9	Class I obesity
35-39.9	Class II obesity
40-49.9	Class III obesity
50-59.9	Super obese
> 60	Super, super obese

Circumference Measurements

The advantage of circumference (girth) measurements is that it is quick and easy and only requires a tape measure that's used to record the circumferences of various body areas. While this information can be plugged into equations to estimate body composition, it's more likely that data will be used to help the trainer/client follow changes in girth over time. For those working with very overweight individuals, this method offers a way to track changes while at the same time not making the client feel overly self-conscious. For a more complete picture of body composition, however, combine it with another method (e.g., skin folds, BIA, etc).

Usually, measurements of upper limb circumferences are taken in the straightened, un-flexed position. This will provide information on the limb's resting girth. Additionally, some may also take measurements of limbs when they are flexed, in order to obtain information about how big a muscle is initially and how much it has developed over time. Normally only the right limbs are measured, if calculating body composition. If possible, remove excess clothing, as this may lead to inaccurate results. Also, a second person may be needed to properly position the measuring tape (e.g., abdomen and hips). When working with very obese people remember that the measuring tape may not be long enough to fully encircle abdominal girth. Those wanting to avoid embarrassing situations may wish to *not* measure this area in very overweight individuals.

Circumference Measurements[3]

Area	Location of Measurement
Neck	At Adam's apple
Shoulder	At maximum bulges of deltoid muscles. Record after normal expiration
Chest	Just above the nipple line. Take measurement after normal expiration.
Waist	At the narrowest part of the waist which is usually above the belly button. Take measurement after normal expiration.
Abdominal	At belly button or at the point of greatest abdominal protuberance
Hip	At the maximum protuberance of the buttocks
Thigh	Largest circumference of thigh, close to buttocks
Calf	At thickest part of calf
Upper Arm (biceps)	At maximum girth of upper arm when arm is relaxed
Forearm	At maximum girth of forearm when arm is relaxed

Abdominal Waist Circumference

Those who carry most of their weight around the belly are at elevated risk of obesity related diseases. Specifically, research indicates that men who have a waist circumference greater than 40 inches (102 cm) and women whose waist is greater than 35 inches (88 cm) are at higher risk of heart disease, type II diabetes, hypertension, high cholesterol and other obesity related issues.[162] Thus, this measurement is important. The measurement is at the narrowest part of the waist, usually a little bit above the belly button, after a normal exhalation. The waist circumference can be especially useful in those who are deemed *normal* or *overweight* by BMI alone. In other words, if the BMI indicates they are "normal" their waist girth may still indicate increased risk of disease.[162] Thus, calculating waist circumference and BMI appear to be better than BMI alone in some people. This may be particularly helpful when dealing with older adults and Asians where waist girth appears to predict disease risk better than BMI.[162] In those whose BMI is over 35, waist circumference usually adds little to the ability to predict overall disease-risk.[162]

Some may also calculate the *waist to hip ratio* (*WHR*). The waist to hip ratio is also used to estimate the degree of abdominal obesity, which indicates risk for heart disease. As the WHR increases, the risk of obesity-related diseases also is increased.[2] A waist to hip ratio greater than 0.95 for adult men or 0.86 for adult women indicates that individuals are at greater risk of developing diseases associated with being overweight.[3] If waist circumference is determined, however, calculating the waist to hip circumference is usually not necessary since it doesn't appear to offer any advantages to waist girth alone.[162]

Waist to Hip Ratio

Male	Female	Health Risk
≤ 0.95	≤ 0.80	Low Risk
0.96 – 1.0	0.81 -0.85	Moderate Risk
≥ 1.0	≥ 0.85	High Risk

Bioelectric Impedance Analysis

Bioelectric impedance analysis (BIA) is very popular in fitness because its quick and easy to administer. Bioelectric impedance analysis works by passing a low intensity electric current through the body and measuring its resistance.[1] Muscle is a better conductor of electricity than fat because of its greater water content. Thus, an electric current will travel slower through a body that has a higher percent body fat. In this way, BIA is able to provide a quick and relatively accurate estimate of body composition. BIA devices usually cost less than $100 and come in hand-held versions and those that a person can stand on. Some models also calculate BMI and still others may have an "athlete mode" which, in theory, may provide a greater degree of accuracy for those who exercise on a regular basis. Whichever type is chosen, the accuracy of BIA, depends on several guidelines:

General BIA Guidelines

1. **Do not** eat or drink for at least four hours before the test
2. **Do not** exercise at least 12 hours before the test
3. **Do** urinate 30 minutes before the test
4. **Do not** drink alcohol at least 48 hours before the test
5. **Do no**t ingest any diuretics (including caffeine) before the test unless prescribed by physician

The equations used today in commercially available machines are probably reasonably accurate for most individuals however, some machines may be unable to determine body composition on those with very high or very low body fat. For example, an error message may result in some machines if used on people who weigh over 300 pounds. Error messages may likewise occur in bodybuilders or others with very low body fat percentages.

BIA may be inappropriate in person's who have pacemakers, defibulators or other implantable heart devices. A possibility exists where the electric current of the BIA device may accidentally set off a pacemaker/defibulator. Fitness professionals should ask everyone, regardless of age, as to whether they have a pacemaker/defibulator. In addition, BIA should not be performed on pregnant women.

Skin Fold Analysis

Skin fold analysis refers to the use of special calipers that essentially *pinch* people at different parts of the body. This method is made possible because a relationship exists between the fat just under the skin (subcutaneous fat) and one's total amount of body fat.[2] Thus, you can estimate total body fat by measuring the fat under the skin. The caliper device measures the thickness of various skin folds. All readings should be taken on the right side of the body only.[3] Also, perform before exercise, never after exercise. This information is then plugged into equations to calculate an estimation of body composition. When performed correctly, the skin fold technique may be accurate to about ± 3% making it very accurate. The operative word is "correctly." This method takes time to learn.

Drawbacks to Skin Fold Testing

1. Total body fat does not just depend on the fat under the skin. Skin fold analysis cannot determine fat around organs.
2. The degree of accuracy depends on the expertise of the person performing the test.
3. Equations for this method are gender, age and race specific. Thus, using the wrong equation will generate a less accurate result.
4. Some people are not comfortable being pinched by people they do not know.
5. This method may not be appropriate for the very overweight.

While, skin fold analysis can be accurate, fitness professionals should remember that new clients may not enjoy being pinched by people they do not know well. Also, some may not enjoy body fat analysis in general. That is, thin people may enjoy seeing their low percentage of body fat while overweight people may not.

Fitness professionals have probably experienced the frustration of people who, after dieting and exercising for weeks, only manage to decrease their body fat by a percentage or two. While this indeed may amount to several pounds of lost fat, seeing a drop of only 1% can be discouraging. Another option is to simply add up all the measurements for each site.[16] In other words, record the areas as you normally do and add them up. Then, several weeks or months later, do the same thing again— record the measurements and add them up. In theory, this second result will be smaller (assuming the person stuck to their workout and eating program). For example:

Site Measured	Measurement (August)*	New Measurement (December)*	Difference (Aug - Dec)
Triceps	11.9	9.7	2.2
Quadriceps	32.5	29.5	3.0
Abs	25.8	22.5	3.3
Suprailiac	14.0	11.0	3.0
Totals	**84.2**	**72.7**	**11.5**

*All measurements in millimeters

In this example you can see that all the measurements taken in August add up to 84.2 millimeters. When the same sites are measured again in December the sites add up to 72.7 mm. This means the person has lost 11.5 mm overall from when the person started (84.2 - 72.5=11.5)! For some, this might be a better method than stating that the person lost 1% of their body fat.

Near Infrared Interactance

The estimation of body composition by near infrared interactance (NIR) makes use of a specialized probe that is placed against an area of the body (e.g., the biceps) which emits infrared light that is passed through muscle and fat. Fat and muscle will absorb and reflect different frequencies of light. The NIR machine then uses this information along with age and activity level to estimate body composition. While variations of this technique have been used in clinical settings since the 1960s, portable devices that are commercially available have been shown to be less accurate than skin fold techniques and bioelectric impedance analysis, described above. Some research finds that NIR might overestimate body fatness in lean people and underestimate it in overweight people.[162] More study is needed before NIR is universally accepted.

Hydrostatic Weighing

Hydrostatic weighing is often called the "gold standard" of body composition analysis because it is one of the most accurate methods and the basis upon which all the others are compared. Because of this, hydrostatic weighing is often used in clinical research. The other name for this is *underwater weighing*, a phrase derived from the fact that people are completely submerged underwater to determine body composition. Hydrostatic weighing is based on *Archimedes's Principle*—that is, a body buoyed in water will be forced to the surface by a force equal to the volume of water that it displaces. In other words, fat floats; the more fat a person has, the lighter they will be when weighted underwater. Usually the person sits on a specialized scale and is completely submerged in water. The individual then forcibly exhales as much air from the lungs as possible and remains motionless. For individuals who are uncomfortable with being submerged under the water as well as those who are not comfortable being in a bathing suit, this method can be a frightening experience. While accurate, underwater weighing needs special equipment and as such is unlikely to be offered in a health club setting.

Air Displacement

Just as hydrostatic weighing measures the displacement of water, body composition can also be determined by measuring the amount of air that a person displaces. The most popular of these types of machines is the Bod Pod®, which measures air displacement when people sit in a special chamber. Clinical studies have been published on the Bod Pod and many find it to be very accurate.[10,11] While body composition can be determined in a matter of minutes, it can cost tens of thousands of dollars, putting it out of reach for many health clubs.

Dual Energy X-Ray Absorptiometry

In addition to its more common use—determining bone density—dual energy x-ray absorptiometry (or *DEXA Scan*) can also precisely estimate the amount of fat and lean muscle tissue that is present. Some consider this method to be more accurate than underwater weighing. That being said, because it uses low level radiation, DEXA is very unlikely to be found at any health club but rather is reserved for hospitals and other clinical research settings.

Estimating Muscle Mass

People sometimes want to know how much muscle is on their body. If you know their percent body fat you can estimate this. For example, suppose someone is 200 lbs and is 20% body fat. 200 X 0.2 = 40 pounds of fat. Subtract this from the total body weight and you get 200 - 40 = 160 pounds of fat-free mass which we typically refer to as muscle. However, this calculation is only an estimate. For example, fat-free mass is not just muscle. Fat-free mass is everything other than fat (hair, water, etc.). Another possible error is the percent body fat. Many techniques (BIA, skin folds, etc.) are not 100% accurate. Failure to adhere to the guidelines of these methods will ramp up inaccuracy.

Additional Tests

In addition to tests of strength, endurance and other areas previously mentioned, it is wise to also measure both resting heart rate and blood pressure. These are important because they may give valuable clues as to the general health of the individual.

Resting Heart Rate

Resting heart rate (RHR) is the number of times a heart beats at rest. We obtain RHR by measuring the pulse which is the sensation we can feel as blood is pumped through the blood vessels. While medical professionals usually take note of the strength of the pulse as well as its rhythm, most others – including fitness professionals – usually just measure the number of beats the heart makes in a minute because it can represent one aspect of general physical fitness.

The average resting heart rate of an adult is 60 to 100bpm.[5] A resting heart rate above 100 bpm is technically classified as *tachycardia* and a resting heart rate below 60 bpm is usually called *bradycardia*. These terms are general and without medical interpretation, don't mean much. In other words, tachycardia could be caused by heart disease, emotional stress, some herbal supplements or simply running up a flight of stairs. By the same token, bradycardia could be caused by some medications (e.g., beta blockers) as well as long-term regular participation in exercise.

Resting Heart Rate and Overtraining Syndrome

Overtraining syndrome represents a series of related issues that tend to occur when a person spends so much time working out that they do not give their body enough time to recover properly. This, in turn, can lead to a decrease in exercise performance. One of the signs of overtraining syndrome is an elevation of resting heart rate. For example, someone with this condition may have a RHR of 85bpm—even though they work out 3 hours a day, 7 days a week! While overtraining syndrome is unlikely in the typical person who exercises, it's a real possibility in athletes, both professional and amateur as well as "gym rats". The only cure for overtraining syndrome is to drastically cut back on the length and intensity of workouts. It may take months before the symptoms subside. Keeping a record of resting heart rate is one of the easiest ways to avoid overtraining syndrome. Other classic signs of this condition include increased infection rate, increase in injuries, insomnia, and decreased exercise performance.

When taking a pulse (especially on another person), it is probably best to do so on the thumb side of the wrist (called the radial pulse) rather than the side of the neck (carotid arteries). This is because there are pressure receptors in the carotid arteries of the neck. Pressing too hard activates these receptors, which, in turn, stimulates a nerve that slows the heart rate.[2] In addition, when taking the pulse, use the index and middle fingers to palpate the area; do not use the thumb. It has its own pulse and this may interfere with your reading.[2] While the best time to obtain RHR is in the morning before people get out of bed, for trainers, having the person sit quietly for 5-10 minutes, will suffice. People should also refrain from smoking or consuming caffeine for at least 30 minutes prior to the test because both of these can elevate heart rate.

When taking a pulse, count the first beat as "one," followed by "two," "three," and so on. Some people choose to take a pulse for an entire minute to obtain RHR. Others may take the pulse for 30 seconds and then multiply the result by 2 (30 x 2 =60 seconds). As a rule, longer time periods are probably best for obtaining RHR while shorter times might be better for determining exercise heart rate. When first learning to take the pulse, take it for a full minute to make sure you counted correctly. Remember, the shorter the time you take the pulse, the greater the error if you miscount. For example, if you're taking a pulse for 6 seconds and you miss a beat, your answer will be off by 10 beats!

In addition to its role in general fitness, some research suggests that heart rate may provide information on long-term health. For example, one study involved 5700 apparently healthy men who were given exercise tests and then followed by researchers for 23 years.[15] Decades after the initial tests, researchers noted that some of the men were at increased risk of sudden death. This observation was seen: 1) in men who had a RHR of more than 75bpm; 2) in men whose heart rate increased by less than 89 bpm during maximal exercise; 3) in men whose heart rate decreased by less than 25 bpm after exercise was stopped. Since long-term exercise (especially aerobic exercise) tends to lower RHR, taking note of a new client's RHR may arm fitness professionals with knowledge that can help people to avoid health problems down the road.

Factors that Impact Heart Rate

When someone takes a heart rate, whether it is upon waking or at another time, they are in effect taking a snapshot of the heart rate at that particular point in time. Heart rate (as well as blood pressure) changes throughout the day. How it changes can depend on a number of environmental, nutritional, emotional and pharmacological factors. For example, many reading these words are well aware that the herbal product, bitter orange, found in some "ephedra free" weight loss supplements can raise heart rate (and blood pressure). Caffeine and smoking likewise can elevate heart rate. Even walking up a flight of steps can significantly alter heart rate (and blood pressure).

Factors That Can Alter Heart Rate

Stimulants (e.g., caffeine)	Some herbs (e.g., bitter orange)
Smoking	Emotional stress
Digestion of food	Age
Position of the body	Time of day
Some medications	Exercise / physical exertion

Notice from the table that some medications can affect heart rate. This may be an issue with some individuals who are taking medications for heart disease. In general, a resting heart rate of 60 bpm or less in older people who do not exercise, may signify that the person is taking heart or blood pressure medication that slows resting heart rate. When encountering these people, it will not be possible to assign a target heart rate range by either the 220 - Age equation or Karvonen equation. Rather, these people are better served by using either the *talk test* or *Borg (RPE) scale*. Heart rate/blood pressure medication usage should also be a red flag to trainers that significant medical issues exist. In this instance, both client and trainer are best served if a written release from the client's physician is obtained prior to training.

Blood Pressure

The blood pressure is the pressure of the blood exerted on the walls of the blood vessels. As the heart beats (contracts), it squeezes blood through the blood vessel system. The pressure of the blood as it is pushed through the blood vessels can be easily measured by essentially listening for sound vibrations (called Korotkoff sounds). All that is needed is a stethoscope and a blood pressure cuff (sphygmomanometer). When the blood pressure cuff is wrapped around the upper arm and is inflated, it eventually cuts off the blood supply. This usually occurs when the cuff is inflated to a pressure of between 180-220 mm Hg (mm Hg is shorthand for *millimeters of Mercury*).

Your blood pressure is actually made up of two separate pressures that are written as a fraction. They are called the *systolic* (pronounced sis-tol-ik) blood pressure (the top number of the fraction) and the *diastolic* (pronounced die-is-tol-ik) blood pressure (the bottom number of the fraction). For example, if your blood pressure was 120/80, 120 is your systolic pressure and 80 is your diastolic pressure. More specifically, the systolic pressure is the blood pressure that results when the heart is contracting, pushing blood out of the heart. Diastolic pressure is the pressure in the blood vessels when your heart is filling with blood, getting ready to contract again.

Blood Pressure Ranges[75]

Normal	Less than 120/80
Prehypertension	120/80 - 139/89
Hypertension	Greater than 140/90

It is not the responsibility of the fitness professional to diagnose hypertension. Only a physician can diagnose a disease/condition. Usually a physician will take several blood pressures before making this determination. Fitness trainers can, though, report abnormal blood pressure to a physician or make this information available to the client so that he/she can do so.

Many people still believe that 120/80 is "normal" however from the table we see that it is not. Less than 120/80 is now normal. A pressure of 120/80 is call called *prehypertension*. This term was invented in 2003 in light of research showing that men over 50 years of age had a 90% chance of developing high blood pressure at some point in their lifetimes if they started out with a BP of 120/80.[17] High blood pressure is often called the "silent killer" because it doesn't have any overt signs or symptoms until it's too late. On prescription pads, physicians will usually abbreviate hypertension as "HTN" or "HBP." The cut off point for high blood pressure is a consistent, resting pressure of at least 140/90.

How to Take Blood Pressure

Blood pressure should be measured in a comfortable, seated position with feet on the floor. Ideally, 5 minutes of rest should precede the test to help normalize blood pressure. The person should not smoke for at least 30 minutes before the test. Supinate the arm so that the palm is facing up. The blood pressure cuff should be wrapped around the upper arm at the level of the heart.[1] The arm should be resting on a table or chair. Either the right or left arm can be used. Because blood pressure can vary slightly between the left and right arms, it may be wise to measure both arms and choose the side that gives the higher readings. Always measure the same arm (and same time of day if possible) when you take blood pressures as this will help produce the most consistent results.

Place the stethoscope over the brachial artery and inflate the cuff to about 180-220 mm Hg or about 20 mm above what their blood pressure usually is. Slowly let the air out of the cuff, taking note to listen for sounds. The first sound you hear will be the systolic blood pressure. The point where you no longer hear any other sound is the diastolic blood pressure. Record these values as the person's blood pressure. For example, if you heard the first sound at 120 mm Hg and ceased to hear sounds at 80 mm Hg, the person's blood pressure is 120/80 mm Hg.

Steps for Taking Successful Blood Pressure Readings[1]

1. People should not smoke or use caffeine for at least 30 minutes before the test
2. Have the person sit quietly for about 5 minutes before the test
3. If the person wears long sleeves that bunch up when rolled up the arm, if possible ask him/her to remove the garment, prior to testing
4. Wrap the blood pressure cuff around the upper arm, at the level of the heart
5. Line up the cuff with the brachial artery
6. The stethoscope should be placed over the brachial artery, located in front of the elbow at the antecubital space
7. Inflate the blood pressure cuff to between 180-220 mm Hg or about 20 mm Hg above what you think their systolic blood pressure is
8. Slowly release the pressure in the cuff and listen for sounds
9. The first sound you hear is the systolic BP. Note the pressure when you no longer hear any sounds. This is the diastolic BP.

When taking blood pressure keep in mind to use the correct blood pressure cuff size. A cuff that is too small can overestimate blood pressure while a cuff that is too big can make blood pressure seem less than it truly is. To determine this first measure the arm circumference with a tape measure. Measure the upper arm midway between the elbow and shoulder.[5] If the circumference is 18-24 cm, use the "child" cuff. For circumferences that are 24-32 cm use the standard "adult" size. Finally, for circumferences of 32-42 cm use the "large adult" cuff.[5] Blood pressure cuffs are sold at most medical/nursing supply stores.

Possible Sources of Error When Testing Blood Pressures[1]

Wrong size cuff	Room noise	Too much pressure on stethoscope
Inability to hear Korotkoff sounds	Inexperience of person giving test	Holding on to treadmill/bike (if testing during exercise)
Improper stethoscope placement	Clenching fists/arms during test	Deflating cuff too fast/slow
Sphygmomometer not calibrated	Stethoscope is used backward	Stethoscope is under BP cuff

> ## Blood Pressure and Exercise
>
> The normal response of blood pressure to aerobic exercise is for the systolic blood pressure to increase as exercise intensity is increased. The diastolic BP will either remain unchanged or may decrease very slightly. Failure of systolic BP to rise as exercise is made harder may be a sign of an emergency. In this case, the heart can't meet the demands of exercise any longer. Repeat the BP test instantly and if you get the same result, stop the exercise test and call 911 immediately.

Types of Blood Pressure Cuffs

The type of blood pressure cuff used mostly in research and clinical settings is the *mercury* cuff. This is the type that is considered the "gold standard" because it is most accurate and does not need to be recalibrated over time. When inflated, a column of mercury rises in a glass chamber.

Another popular sphygmomanometer is the *aneroid* type. This blood pressure cuff is easily recognized because instead of a vertical column of mercury, it has a round dial with a small needle inside. As the cuff is inflated, the needle moves to greater pressures. While popular, this type may need to be recalibrated over time. Occasionally, readings with aneroid blood pressure cuffs should be compared to those obtained with the more accurate mercury-filled versions.

Electronic versions of blood pressure cuffs are also available to the public. These machines inflate automatically and take blood pressure with just the touch of a button. While they may have merit in some situations, they may not be as accurate as either mercury or aneroid blood pressure cuffs for all individuals and should not be used in place of seeing a physician regularly. Some portable types measure blood pressure around the wrist. This may lead to additional points of error.

Recognizing a Heart Attack

Because heart disease is the number one killer of Americans (stroke is the number 3 killer), it is possible that at some point the fitness professional may have to render CPR or utilize an AED in the event a heart attack occurs. A heart attack may occur at any time, ranging from resting to fitness testing or after years of working out. Regardless, recognizing the warning signs of a heart attack or stroke can help minimize the effects of such an occurrence.

Signs of a Heart Attack[89]

1. **Chest pain or discomfort.** The chest pain or discomfort can last for as little as 3-5 minutes or go away and return later. The pain can be perceived as a squeezing of the chest or just an uncomfortable feeling.
2. **Pain elsewhere on upper body.** Heart attack pain may also be felt in the jaw, stomach, back or in one or both arms.
3. **Shortness of breath.** This may or may not accompany chest pain.
4. **Other symptoms.** Less common symptoms of a heart attack can be sweating, light-headedness or nausea/vomiting.

In addition to chest pain or discomfort, according to the American Heart Association, women may be more likely to complain of other symptoms like shortness of breath, nausea/vomiting or pain in the jaw or back.[89]

Stroke Warning Signs[88]

1. Sudden numbness/weakness in the face, arm or leg — especially limited to one side of the body.
2. Sudden confusion or trouble speaking or understanding.
3. Sudden trouble seeing out of one or both eyes.
4. Sudden trouble walking, dizziness, loss of coordination or balance.
5. Sudden severe headache with no known cause.

Coming face to face with a heart attack or stroke can be a traumatic experience and it is normal to be afraid. This is why it is imperative that all fitness professionals have a current CPR and AED certification. During this situation it is important that you remain calm and if you work in a health club, follow the health club's emergency procedures.

Chapter 12

GETTING A JOB IN FITNESS

One of the most frequent questions asked by people just starting out is how to go about obtaining their first job. It is here, at your first job, that you will learn many of the crucial skills that will ultimately shape you as you grow in the field. While knowing what aspect of fitness you want to specialize in (kids fitness, seniors, etc.) is important, most have no idea of this when they are first starting out. Rather, most are just looking to get their feet wet and see where it takes them. This chapter is included to help give you the advice and tools you will need to land a job — and make a lasting impression.

Where Will You Work?

Even if your ultimate goal is to go in to business for yourself, you will probably start out by working for someone else. For many, this means working in a fitness center. This is actually a pretty good place to start because gives you the opportunity to familiarize yourself with a wide range of exercise equipment. This information can help you years later if you are asked by future clients to recommend equipment for their homes. You also have the opportunity to learn other aspects of the fitness business like sales, the front desk, manager responsibilities and equipment maintenance, to name a few. If you work in a health club, it is in your long-term best interest to expose yourself to as much about the organization as possible. What you learn now will serve you in the future.

Advantages of Working in a Fitness Center

Exposure to wide range of fitness equipment	Interaction with many different types of people	Learning from others
Making business contacts	Potential to move up the corporate ladder	Learning how to deal with various types of people
Management training	Opening / closing procedures	Front desk operations

Many times, getting an interview may be as easy as walking in the front door of a club and asking for either the *Fitness Director*, *GM* or *Manager on Duty* (MOD). These are the people who generally have the ability to hire or are in a position to get you an interview. Sometimes you may be asked to complete an application on the spot, while other times they may make you return at a future date for the interview. When in doubt, however, it's good to be prepared.

When looking for a job, it's a good idea to survey several fitness centers before you actually apply for a position. That way, you'll know in advance what each has to offer. Also, feel free to apply to several positions at once. This reduces the chances that you will be *behind the eight ball*, waiting for a single perspective employer to call you back.

Interviewing for a Job

Interviewing for a job can be stressful but it doesn't have to be, because it is not only *they* who are interviewing you but *you* who are interviewing them! This is your time to ask questions and determine if they suit your needs. Before the interview take note of these tips to help you make a lasting impression.

1. *Bring your resume with you.* Your resume doesn't have to be fancy or have industry-specific experience. In your resume, you should list your fitness certifications, CPR/AED certs, college degrees or other educational experience, internships, previous fitness related experience, fitness-related interests and any related skills you feel would help the company. If you have competed in the Ironman Triathlon, climbed Mt. Everest or took part in any fitness-related event, include this also. If you are brand new to the industry, don't worry if you do not have much experience. The fact that you present a resume will speak volumes about your character and professionalism! Don't worry if you have never created a resume either. They are easy to do. There are books on how to write a resume that you can find at bookstores or libraries. Sample resumes can also be found online. Bring your resume to the interview in a padfolio for safe keeping. Carry it in your left hand so you can easily shake hands with people. The padfolio should have paper and pencil available so that you can take notes during the interview. This is also a place for you to write the questions you have about the job for which you are interviewing. Write these questions down before the interview. This says to employers that you are taking the position seriously.

2. *Dress appropriately for the interview.* Generally, fitness is a casual field, so dressing up in a suit and tie is usually not necessary (unless you are interviewing for a management or GM position, in which case it is). Usually khakis, casual shoes and a polo shirt are sufficient for most fitness job interviews. Dressing for the interview says to management that you're a mature person and take the interview seriously. This elevates you over all others who don't dress up.

3. *After the interview, send a thank-you letter.* A thank-you letter is a common courtesy in business and should be mailed a day or two after the interview. Just a short letter thanking the person for their time is all that's needed. Generally, handwritten notes are more personal than those that are typed on a computer. The letter demonstrates to the employer that you appreciate the time they spent interviewing you. Do include your phone number and address to make it easier for the person doing the hiring to reach you. Most people in fitness probably will not send a thank-you note, so this is another excellent way for you to stand out in the eyes of management. Even if you do not get the job you want, the odds are very good that management will remember your name and if an opening occurs in the future, you probably will be first on their list to contact.

Interview Questions

During the interview you will be asked questions so that the organization can get to know you better. Here is a list of very common questions you may be asked during an interview. It is suggested that you review these questions and think about your answers ahead of time.

Possible Interview Questions

1. Why do you want to work for us? (Probably the most common question asked!)
2. Where do you see yourself in 5 or 10 years?
3. What do you feel are your strengths?
4. What do you feel are your weaknesses?
5. Why should we hire you for this job?
6. Do you prefer to work alone or as part of a team?
7. Give an example of a difficult situation you faced and how you resolved it.
8. Why did you leave your most recent job?
9. How would you describe your style of management?
10. What would you say is the biggest difference between us and your previous employer?

Questions You Should Ask During an Interview

A job interview is not just for the employer to ask you questions. Rather, it's a time for you to ask questions too! By asking questions of your potential employer you send a strong message that you have done your homework about their organization. A good place to start is at the company's website.

Possible Questions to Ask During an Interview

1. How many members does the club currently have?
2. What is the average age of the clubs members?
3. What organizations are the fitness staff certified by?
4. What is the fitness philosophy of the health club?
5. What are the duties/responsibilities of the position for which I am interviewing?
6. Are there any skills that you feel are crucial to success in the position?
7. How will my job performance be measured and by whom?
8. Does the club provide any educational incentives to help me advance my knowledge?
9. Is there room for growth within the organization?
10. What are the established procedures to follow in the event of a medical emergency?

This last question, asking about emergency procedures, I feel is particularly important given that accidents – minor and serious – do occur from time to time in health clubs. Having a competent staff makes a manager's job easier. Nowhere is this more important than in an emergency situation. Also, you may be the only one who has ever asked this question, which again sets you apart from the rest of the pack in the eyes of the management.

Interview Mistakes

Years ago, I applied for a job in telemarketing. During the interview I was asked the dreaded question, "Why do you want to work for us?" to which I replied confidently, "Because it's easy!" Needless to say, I didn't get the job. Truth be told, the job was easy compared to my last job where I washed dishes in a hot kitchen for so long that the skin flaked off my hands! The person interviewing me didn't care that I left for the interview at 6AM and took two buses in the pouring rain to be on time for the interview. In her mind, all she heard was that I didn't take the job seriously. To make sure your interview goes well, never say the job is "easy" and follow these additional tips.

Tips for a Great Interview

1. Show up on time for the interview.
2. Turn your cell phone off. If your phone rings during the interview don't answer it.
3. Do bring your resume and dress appropriately.
4. Do not talk badly about former employers during the interview.
5. Do maintain eye contact when speaking.
6. Be friendly yet professional during the interview.
7. Do know about the company ahead of time – check their website.
8. Do mirror the demeanor of the interviewer. If he/she is all business, you be all business too.
9. Do mention your strengths and how they would fit with the organization.
10. Do be enthusiastic about the job for which you are interviewing.

How Much Is The Salary?

At some point during the interview the salary of the position will probably be raised by the person doing the hiring. While some feel it's rude for the interviewee to ask about salary, I do not – especially if the issue is not brought up by the time the interview is almost over.

With respect to fitness trainers, salary is usually composed of an hourly wage plus commissions. The hourly wage will vary but is generally $6-$20 per hour for "floor time"–the time fitness trainers are in the fitness center, helping members and trying to get clients. Commissions are where fitness trainers usually make most of their money. Generally, personal training and fitness commissions range from 40%-65% of the amount paid to the club. For example, if a member paid $50 for a personal training session and the trainer was getting a 50% commission, he/she would make $25 for that session. While personal training sessions may last 60 minutes, some clubs cut it back to 30 to 45 minutes. This allows the fitness trainer to do more sessions per day and make more money.

Some health clubs may pay different commission rates based on your education, years experience, etc. This sometimes leads to titles like "Level One Trainer" "Master Trainer" etc. Clubs generally want to hold onto good personal trainers and they tend to reward those who continue to sharpen their skills.

Chapter 13

QUESTIONS AND ANSWERS

For years I've been getting emails from people all over the world who are looking for honest answers to their fitness questions. Here are some of those questions. The following were chosen because they give you a glimpse into the types of questions people will ask you as a personal trainer; hopefully also they will help reinforce the need for fitness trainers to stay educated.

Q. What precautions should female trainers take before going to the home of a new client?

A. Because of the internet it's sometimes possible to discover information about the client before meeting with him/her. Checking your area's sex offender registry website may also help. At least one friend should know the location of all client's names and addresses. Trainers should also carry a cell phone with them and call a friend/significant other just prior to entering a client's home, especially if they do not know the person. Many cell phones can now be tracked via GPS. They should tell the friend the name and address of the client they are meeting, as well as the start and end times of the session and call that friend again when the session ends. Some trainers will make a point to mention during the session that they have an appointment immediately after the meeting so that the client knows the trainer is expected elsewhere and even let the client see them talking on the phone when the client opens the door. Some women may also carry pepper spray or other personal defense items. Women should be suspicious of people who want to meet at night or at secluded locations or who make strange requests. Never feel pressured to meet someone if you don't feel comfortable while talking to that person on the phone. Technically both men and women should take precautions like this because, unfortunately, the world is not as safe as it used to be.

Q. I am a female trainer and one of my clients is sexually harassing me. What can I do?

A. You may want to pass the client along to another trainer. You should also discuss the matter with the club's general manager and let the GM take appropriate action against the offending club member. It's also wise to document all occurrences of the harassment, noting the dates and times of the incidents, witnesses, and as many specifics as you can recall. Copies of the incidents should go to the GM and you should also retain copies for your own records. The gym is obligated to provide a safe, environment for its employees. This includes being free from sexual harassment from the club's members and other staff. The GM should keep you in the loop as to the action he/she took to deal with the problem. If the harassment continues, you have other legal options which an attorney can best provide for you. The same procedure also applies to men who are sexually harassed.

Q. What might cause a person to feel a burning sensation in their calves when they start walking? It stops soon after they sit down. What is this?

A. While personal trainers can't really determine for certain, a burning or cramping sensation in the calves, felt soon after physical activity could be a sign of *intermittent claudication*, which may indicate peripheral artery disease (PAD). These are linked to heart disease. This condition results in a lack of blood flow to the legs due to the buildup of artery-clogging plaque. Sometimes the pain is felt in the thighs or buttocks also. Typically the sensation starts after a few minutes of walking and stops soon after ceasing the activity. Because other factors may also cause this condition, people with this complaint should be referred to their physician who can properly diagnose the problem.

Q. Are squats bad for the knees?

A. Several studies have found that squats are not innately harmful to the knees.[131] In fact, it is the official position of the National Strength and Conditioning Association (NSCA) that if performed correctly, squats may even help reduce knee injuries by helping to stabilize the knee joint and the muscles around that joint.[131] It is interesting to note that the original research on this dates back to the 1960s and was actually referring to deep squats, which go below 90°. It is also noteworthy that the deep knee squatting research has since been criticized by other investigators.[131] Nevertheless, more research is needed before this controversy is fully resolved.[185]

Q. How much exercise do people need?

A. Generally speaking, people should strive for between 30 to 60 minutes moderate intensity (e.g., 3-6 METs) of physical activity most day of the week.[1] Thirty minutes is thought, by some, to be the *minimum* amount of exercise needed to maintain general health. Also, the activity does not all have to be obtained at the same time. For example, two 15 minute exercise sessions appears to be as good as a single 30 minute session. Some guidelines for losing weight call for up to 90 minutes of activity most days of the week.

Q. Do heavier people have slower metabolisms?

A. While possible, this is generally false. Heavier people and taller people tend to have higher resting metabolic rates than thinner and shorter people.

Q. Are natural vitamins better than synthetic vitamins?

A. No. In fact, in some instances, synthetic vitamins are superior. Those who thought that natural vitamins were better are highly encouraged to read my book, *Nutrition Essentials,* which is all about nutrition and sports nutrition and was written specifically for fitness professionals. My other books, *Health and Wellness Q & A* and *Nutritional Supplements* are also an excellent resources. All can be obtained at my website, www.Joe-Cannon.com.

Q. How can I tell the difference between muscle soreness and a more serious pain?

A. Muscle soreness (DOMS) is not felt when the muscle is not moving. This pain usually subsides after several days. On the other hand, feeling pain when the affected area is not moving is a sign of something more serious that should be checked out by a physician.

Q. What's the difference between a sprain and a strain?

A. A strain is an injury to a muscle or tendon (which connects muscles to bones) while a sprain is an injury to a ligament (which connects bones to each other). An easy way to remember the difference is to keep in mind that the word strain contains the letter T (for tendon). A sprain is more of an acute injury while a strain can be acute or occur after repeated trauma (chronic). Both types of injuries are common to people who exercise. Acute versions of both may be helped with RICE (rest, ice, compression, elevation) but more severe types may require physical therapy or other medical interventions.

Q. What's better: ice or heat after an injury?

A. Immediately following an injury, ice is usually the best choice because it helps reduce pain and swelling. Generally, ice is applied 10-15 minutes at a time. This helps reduce frostbite from occurring. Ice can also help some long-term injuries (e.g., tennis elbow). As for heat, if the injury is long-term (chronic), heat can help also because it eases stiff areas. Heat should not be applied right after injury because it can increase swelling. When in doubt, if the injury is not feeling better after a day or two, it's best to see a physician.

Q. Which is better: strength training *before* cardio or cardio *before* strength training?

A. Interestingly, there is little research on this topic. Intuitively, it makes sense that whichever you do first depends primarily on your fitness goals. If your goal is to get stronger, do the strength first. If your goal is to run a marathon, it might be best to do the cardio first. You can also look at this from a metabolic point of view. For example, which sequence elevates metabolic rate (i.e. calorie burning) the most? This may be of interest to people striving for weight loss. One study noted that performing cardio *before* strength training resulted in a slightly greater elevation in metabolic rate (EPOC) than when strength training was performed first.[79] This doesn't mean that performing cardio first is always better. Remember, the body "knows" the order of the exercises it does. It knows the exercise sequence, the weight lifted, the machines used, the speed of the lifts and the rest periods between sets. When it performs the same activity regularly, the body becomes more efficient (i.e., burns fewer calories). So, for those who are seeking weight loss and performing strength training first, try doing cardio first. A month or so later, switch it again. This will keep your body guessing and maximize progress and calorie usage.

Q. Will lifting weights before doing cardio cause the body to burn off its glycogen reserves, and help people burn fat better?

A. Weightlifting before cardio probably does not speed up the fat burning process if you are accustomed to that sequence of exercise. The primary fuel that the body uses during exercise (both strength and cardio) is fat and carbs. The average human body has enough energy in the form of glycogen (carbs) to keep you running for about 20 miles! People just can't burn off that much glycogen by lifting weights for an hour or so. This is actually a good thing because the fat burning process needs carbs to work! Just as a fire needs oxygen to burn, fat needs carbs to burn.

Q. Does muscle weigh more than fat?

A. Technically, muscle does *not* weigh more than fat. A pound of muscle and a pound of fat weigh one pound! Muscle is, *denser* than fat and this is where the confusion stems from. Because it's denser, muscle takes up less space. Muscle also tends to burn more calories than fat. Various studies put the usage at about 20-100 calories per pound of muscle. Fat, on the other hand, uses much fewer calories per pound. So, while they don't technically weigh the same, there are significant differences between muscle and fat.

Q. Can we turn fat into muscle?

A. No. They are two different types of tissues. You can't change one into another.

Q. Can forced reps help weightlifter's increase strength?

A. Forced repetitions occur when the lifter has help performing additional reps after he/she can no longer perform reps on his/her own. One study of basketball and volleyball players who trained for six weeks, found that forced reps did not increase strength any more than when players lifted until muscular failure set in.[126] However, the limited amount of research on this topic makes drawing definitive conclusions about this practice difficult. Because forced reps carry a higher risk of injury, examine its usefulness within the context of a client's health and goals before using.

Q. How does testosterone improve strength?

A. It appears that testosterone not only improves muscle protein synthesis but at the same time slows protein breakdown. One study noted that heavy strength training improved muscle protein synthesis by 50% after 4 hours of exercise and 109% 24 hours later![110] To naturally boost testosterone levels with resistance training it is generally necessary to use heavier loads (e.g., 85% 1RM), coupled with short rest periods and moderate volumes (at least 4 sets). Obviously, this is an advanced protocol and not appropriate for beginners.

Q. Can muscles get stronger without growing larger?

A. Its possible. Remember that muscle hypertrophy and muscle strength do not always go hand-in-hand and it is possible for muscles to grow stronger without a corresponding increase in muscle size. This appears to be especially true in prepubescent children, women and in those who have worked out for at least two years.[109]

Q. Is there a difference between weight bearing exercise and weightlifting?

A. Yes. Weight bearing activity occurs when you are supporting ("bearing") your weight. Walking, for example, is a weight bearing activity (but water walking or water aerobics are not). Also, if you are sitting, you are not weight bearing. Weight lifting, on the other hand, is moving an external resistance through a range of motion. Both can help strengthen bones, but since weight bearing usually involves the lower body, it tends to do little for the muscles and bones of the upper body.

Q. How much protein do exercisers need?

A. The best research available suggests that most people who exercise regularly can make gains in strength by using 1.2-1.8 g/kg/BW which is about 0.6-0.9 grams per pound.[72,182] Those who do primarily cardio should stay at the lower end while those who primarily strength train may benefit from the higher end of this range. The often repeated mantra of "1 gram per pound" for everybody has no basis in scientific fact. For more sports nutrition facts, read my book *Nutrition Essentials*, available at my website www.Joe-Cannon.com.

Q. When using creatine supplements, is the "loading phase" needed?

A. The loading phase typically consists of taking 20 or so grams of creatine per day for a week, followed by a *maintenance phase* of 2-5 grams per day. One interesting study noted one month of using just 3 grams per day loaded muscles with as much creatine as did a week of using 20 grams per day.[80] Thus, according to this report, the loading phase may not be needed. The loading phase will quickly improve creatine storage and improve muscle power, but if you're not in a hurry, you probably don't need it.

Q. Do creatine supplements have any side effects?

A. The most consistently observed side effect is a gain in water weight. People tend to gain several pounds after a couple of weeks of using creatine supplements. Other side effects, like kidney and liver damage as well as muscle and tendon tears have not been observed in well-designed clinical studies.

Q. Is creatine safe for kids?

A. Children are not miniature adults and may not respond the same as adults to creatine supplementation. Currently there are no large scale reliable studies of creatine supplements in humans under the age of legal consent. Thus, creatine supplements are not recommended for those under 18.

Q. Does caffeine neutralize the power-enhancing properties of creatine?

A. There is some evidence which finds that caffeine might neutralize the power-enhancing effect of creatine supplements.[81,82] According to some research this effect may be related to caffeine extending the relaxation time of muscles before they can contract again.[82] Additionally, this effect of caffeine appears to be greatest when its used a few days prior to exercise but not if used one hour before exercise.[82] Strength and power athletes who supplement with creatine may want to avoid caffeine for several days prior to competition, just to be safe. Read my book *Nutritional Supplements: What Works and Why* for more information on creatine and over 100 other supplements.

Q. Is there any benefit to stretching between sets?

A. Yes. Stretching or performing light aerobic exercise between sets can enhance the clearance of lactic acid and other metabolites from muscles, allowing them to recover faster. This can result in more energetic and forceful muscle contractions on subsequent sets.

Q. What's better for lowering blood pressure: high or low intensity exercise?

A. When it comes to blood pressure, lower intensity exercise (RPE 2-3) tends to do a better job than higher intensity activity.

Q. How can a person have a low resting heart rate if they don't exercise regularly?

A. Usually, RHR decreases when people workout frequently. However, it may also be low when people are using various medications (e.g., beta blockers) used to treat high blood pressure or heart disease.

Q. Why is it that a person can ride a bicycle for 60 miles yet not be able to run 1 mile?

A. It sounds like they have great aerobic capacity but this is not the only factor to consider. Biking works the muscles differently than running. For one thing, running is weight bearing while biking is not. Remember the SAID principle: the body responds specifically to the exercise demands imposed on it. In other words, to be a better runner, don't bike – run!

Q. Are "low fat" foods, healthy?

A. Not necessarily. Because of current laws, it's possible for foods displaying the "low fat" label to contain a lot of fat. To determine if a low fat food really is really low in fat, divide the total calories of the food by the calories from fat and multiply by 100.

Q. Can vitamin C reduce muscle soreness?

A. There is very little evidence that vitamin C or other antioxidants reduce DOMS-related pain.[121] The best defense against DOMS is to progress slowly, starting with one set per exercise.

Q. Can we only absorb nutrients if they are in certain combinations?

A. Claims of this or that special combinations of foods can lead to weight loss are not based on fact. Your body is perfectly able to absorb the nutrients from any combination of foods you eat.

Q. Does exercise increase lactic acid production in breast milk?

A. Usually, expectant mothers who exercise want to know this answer. Generally low to moderate type exercise does not elevate lactic acid levels in breast milk. While intense exercise may, in some instances, slightly raise lactic acid levels, this does not appear to impact the baby's taste for breast milk.[106]

Q. Any advice for a person just starting out in the fitness field who feels intimidated?

A. Don't feel scared. We all have strengths and weaknesses. The more you read, study and work with people, the more you add to your knowledge base — and the more you can help others. Eventually, you will find your niche—the area of fitness you choose to focus on. You will be a better personal trainer after one year than you will be after a month; after 5 years, you'll be even better! If your main rule is "first, do no harm," you will be ok. As Leonard Da Vinci once said, *all obstacles yield to stern resolve.* Focus on your craft and learn all you can. You will never know everything— and that's ok. It's always nice when you learn something new, even after years of study. It keeps us humble and stops us from taking ourselves too seriously.

Q. Where can I get more answers?

A. Go to www.Joe-Cannon.com and download my e-book *Health and Wellness Q & A* which answers well over 135 essential exercise, nutrition and health questions that all people should know. At my website you will also find additional helpful information.

Chapter 14

Special Populations

High Blood Pressure Guidelines

Key Points

➢ Also called hypertension. Defined as a consistent resting blood pressure of at least 140-90.
➢ Prehypertension is a BP of 120/80 (this used to be called "normal").
➢ High blood pressure is a major risk factor for stroke – the 3rd leading cause of death.
➢ BP (especially systolic) tends to increase with age; however, all people should strive to maintain BP below 120/80.[164]
➢ Most cases have no known cause and are called idiopathic or primary hypertension. If the condition can be traced to another factor (obesity, etc.) it is called secondary hypertension.
➢ Not all cases can be controlled by diet and exercise alone.
➢ The following all increase risk: excess body weight, excess dietary sodium, reduced physical activity, and lack of fruits and vegetables in the diet.[164]
➢ Abbreviated as HTN by physicians.

General Guidelines for Hypertension[164]

➢ Lose weight if necessary. Strive for a BMI of 18.5-24.9.
➢ Stop smoking. Reduce saturated fat and cholesterol from diet.
➢ Sodium intake: no more than a teaspoon per day (2300 mg).
➢ Increase potassium-rich foods (fruits and vegetables). Eat according to the DASH eating plan. DASH stands for Dietary Approaches to Stop Hypertension and is available online. DASH emphasis fruits, vegetables and low fat-dairy and reduces saturated fat, total fat and cholesterol intake.
➢ Alcohol. Men: No more than 2 drinks per day. Women: No more than 1 drink per day.
➢ Exercise. Aim for at least 30 minutes of exercise most days of the week.

General Exercise Guidelines[141]

Type of Exercise	Exercise Guideline	Frequency, Intensity, Time
Aerobic	Large-muscle activities	RPE: 2-4 (0-10 scale) 30-60 min per day 3-7 day/wk Aim for burning 700-2000 calories per week
Strength Training	Circuit training	Low resistance, higher number of reps (e.g., 15-20RM)

Comments & Suggestions

➢ If possible, take BP before and after exercise to gauge how exercise impacted BP.

➢ Don't exercise if BP is ≥ 200/115.

➢ Use Borg scale or talk test to gauge exercise intensity if client is on meds that slow heart rate

➢ Weight training should not be the only type of exercise performed.

➢ Use overhead lifts with caution (because of Valsalva maneuver).

➢ Avoid static contractions when possible.

➢ Avoid tight gripping of fitness equipment (e.g., treadmill).

➢ Avoid fast transfers from seated/supine positions to standing.

➢ Lower intensity exercise is better at lowering HTN than higher intensity exercise.

➢ For more information visit the National Heart Lung and Blood Institute www.nhlbi.nih.gov.

High Cholesterol Guidelines

Key Points

- Hyperlipidemia refers to elevated levels of cholesterol and triglycerides.
- Hypercholesterolemia refers specifically to elevated levels of cholesterol (>200 mg/dl).
- Hypertriglyceridemia refers specifically to elevated levels of triglycerides (>150 mg/dl).
- HDL refers to high density lipoprotein (good cholesterol). ≥40 mg/dl is appropriate.
- LDL refers to low density lipoprotein (bad cholesterol). < 100 mg/dl is appropriate.
- VLDL: Very low lipoprotein density. A type of LDL that has the most triglyceride. Normal levels range from 5-40 mg/dl.[175] As triglycerides lower, so, too, does VLDL.[175]
- Elevated levels of LDL, cholesterol and triglycerides are a risk factor for CAD.

General Exercise Guidelines

Type of Exercise	Exercise Guideline	Frequency, Intensity, time
Aerobic	Multi-joint activities	4-6 day per wk/ 40 min per session. RPE 2-4 (0-10 scale) or 11-16 (6-20 scale)
Strength Training	Circuit training	Light weights (e.g., 40%-60% 1 RM) higher reps (e.g.,8-12 reps per set)

Comments & Suggestions

- Weight loss often can lower cholesterol and blood lipid levels.
- The optimal amount of exercise needed to impact lipids may vary from person to person. The main goal is to burn calories during exercise. Because cardio often burns more calories than strength training, it is often emphasized.
- An HDL of 60 mg/dl or more is a "negative risk factor" for heart disease (i.e., it lowers the risk). Exercise— esp. cardio —often ramps up HDL.
- If the person is using beta blockers or other medications that lower RHR, RPE and/or Talk Test are better than HR calculations when estimating exercise intensity.
- Determining 1RM may not be needed or advisable in this population because of other medical issues the person may also have.
- Some dietary supplements may help improve lipid levels naturally. For more information on this topic, read *Nutritional Supplements: What Works and Why*, available at my website, www.Joe-Cannon.com
- Adding a cardio station to the strength training circuit ramps up the aerobic component of the circuit.
- Besides exercise, it's important to limit dietary fat and cholesterol.
- For more information visit the National Heart Lung and Blood Institute www.nhlbi.nih.gov.

Post Heart Attack Guidelines

Key Points

- Technically called myocardial infarction and abbreviated as "MI" by doctors.
- Coronary artery disease can lead to a heart attack and is often abbreviated as "CAD" by doctors.
- Heart attacks result when heart muscle dies from inadequate oxygen supply. This can result when artery-clogging plaque builds up in blood vessels.

General Exercise Guidelines[141]

Type of Exercise	Exercise Guideline	Frequency, Intensity, time
Aerobic	Multi-joint movements	3-4 days per week/ RPE 2-6 (11-16 if using 6-20 scale), 20-40 min per session
Strength Training	Circuit training	2-3 days per week/ 1-3 sets of 10-15 reps

Comments & Suggestions

- People should be evaluated by their physician prior to starting an exercise program. Fitness trainers should obtain written permission from the physician with any instructions prior to training.
- Doctors may quantify exercise capacity in terms of METs. Those with low fitness levels will probably be prescribed an exercise level of 5 METs or less.[141]
- Both warm-up and cool-down periods of about 10 minutes each are essential and may help stabilize heart rate before and after exercise.
- With respect to resistance training, the loads lifted should be light to moderate (e.g., 10-15 reps/ exercise).
- Some training recommendations call for starting a resistance training program at 50% 1RM, however, this usually requires determining 1RM which may not be appropriate.[177] Estimating 1RM from tables may likewise be inappropriate also with this population.[177]
- Begin with only 1 set per exercise.
- When increasing weights, 2-5 lbs for upper body exercises and 5-10 lbs for lower body may be appropriate, but can vary according to fitness level, age, and other health issues.[177]
- Rest periods between sets are generally 1.5-2 minutes, but can vary according to fitness level.[177]
- Remember to remind the person to breathe during resistance training. This stabilizes BP due to the Valsalva maneuver.
- Rising too fast from the seated, supine or prone positions may result in a drop in BP that can lead to fainting (orthostatic hypotension). Supervise when the person rises.
- People may have other issues to consider (e.g., diabetes, overweight etc.) when developing the exercise program.

- If the person is taking beta blockers or other medications that slow HR, The Borg scale is superior to heart rate when monitoring exercise intensity.[141]
- People who have had one heart attack, may be at risk of another one. Be familiar with the signs of a heart attack and remember that high intensity exercise increases this risk.
- People who complain of pain in their ankles or legs upon walking, only to have it subside after ceasing the activity, may have peripheral artery disease (abbreviated as PAD or PVD). Stationary bicycle or upper body aerobic exercise (e.g., UBE) may be an option for these individuals.
- For more information visit the American Heart Association at www.americanheart.org.

Diabetes Guidelines

Key Points

- Diabetes is defined as a metabolic disorder characterized as either a failure to make the hormone insulin (type I) – or the inability to use the insulin that is made (type II). Most cases of diabetes are type II. Type I diabetics must inject insulin to survive. Both genetics and environmental factors play roles in the development of both types.
- Insulin is made in the beta cells of the pancreas. Insulin helps the body use sugar (glucose).
- Normal blood sugar is <100 mg/dl.
- Hemoglobin A1c: A marker of blood sugar levels over the last 3 months.
- Type II diabetes appears to result from problems with insulin receptors. Lack of insulin receptors reduces the ability of insulin to work. Thus, without insulin receptors the body becomes "insulin resistant." That is, they make insulin but are resistant to its effects.
- Type II diabetes may progress to type I if not treated
- Type I diabetes is caused by an autoimmune disorder. The immune system attacks the beta cells which make insulin. This decreases/shuts down insulin production. The reasons why the immune system attacks the beta cells is unknown.
- Metabolic Syndrome. Cluster of conditions that increase risk for type II diabetes (and heart disease). Symptoms include abdominal obesity, reduced HDL, increased LDL and triglycerides, insulin resistance, increased blood pressure. Elevated CRP levels sometimes also noted. Exercise can improve metabolic syndrome.
- Diabetes may be accompanied by heart disease, vision problems, kidney problems, balance problems and hypertension, to name a few.
- Hypoglycemia. Low blood sugar. Signs can include rapid heart rate, sweating, anxiety, tremors, mental confusion and ultimately loss of consciousness.
- Ketosis. Abnormal elevation in ketones. Results from burning the fat without the presence of carbs (glucose). Ketosis upsets acid/base balance of body. If not treated, can lead to death.

General Guidelines for Diabetes

- Lose weight if needed. Even modest weight loss can help. Regular physical activity.
- Maintain appropriate blood sugar levels through proper nutrition, exercise and drug therapy.

General Exercise Guidelines

Type of Exercise	Exercise Guideline	Frequency, Intensity, Time
Aerobic	Use large muscle groups	50%-90% HR max, 20-60 min per session. Most days of week.
Strength training	Interval training. Machines, free weights or combination.	No official guidelines. Use caution with high intensity activity.
Flexibility	Improve balance. Improve flexibility of joints.	No official guidelines

Comments & Suggestions

➤ Don't exercise if blood sugar is >300 mg/dl.

➤ Client should be aware of the different types of insulin and when they are most effective at lowering blood sugar and avoid workouts when the insulin they are using is most effective.

➤ Holding breath during strength training may damage already weakened blood vessels.

➤ If possible measure blood sugar before and after exercise to gauge how exercise impacted blood sugar levels – especially when starting a new exercise program.

➤ Because balance and vision problems are common, stay with client at all times.

➤ Have carbohydrate snacks handy in case blood sugar dips too low.

➤ Remind client that hypoglycemia may occur hours after the workout. Avoid exercising the area of the body that was injected with insulin.

➤ If diabetic passes out, it's safest to give the person sugar (carbs). If hypoglycemia is why the person passed out and insulin is administered, blood sugar will go even lower – which can be fatal.

➤ Increase exercise intensity gradually if athletic performance is a goal. Remember that higher intensities of exercise may increase blood sugar.

➤ Loss of feeling in the feet (neuropathy) can lead to balance problems. Because of lack of feeling, injuries to the feet (blisters, broken bones etc.) may not be noticed.

➤ For more information visit the American Diabetes Association www.diabetes.org.

Arthritis Guidelines

Key Points

- There are over 100 conditions classified as arthritis. The most common type is osteoarthritis. Another common type is rheumatoid arthritis.
- Osteoarthritis (OA or DJD) results from a wearing away of the joint cartilage. Can be caused by injury, ballistic sports participation or obesity. Genetic link is possible also.
- Rheumatoid arthritis (RA) is thought to result from an autoimmune disorder where immune cells attack the joints.
- Both OA and DJD result in deformity of the joints. The areas affected with arthritis will be weaker.

General Exercise Guidelines

Type of Exercise	Exercise Guideline	Frequency, Intensity, time
Aerobic	Mulit-joint movements	3-5 days per wk/ RPE 2-6 / 5-30 min per day
Strength Training	Circuit training	2-3 days per week/ 2-12 reps. Intensity varies with pain levels.

Comments & Suggestions

- People often confuse osteoarthritis with osteoporosis.
- Because arthritis reduces mobility, people may also have osteoporosis as well. Diabetes may also occur.
- Many will be deconditioned, requiring low levels of exercise at first. Thus, starting with light weights and very low reps (e.g., 2) may be warranted for strength training.
- Avoid high repetition, high impact activities and those that use high levels of resistance.
- Activates that focus on balance, walking and ADLs may help improve quality of life.
- Stretching is important to maintain pain-free ROM; however overstretching joints may exacerbate pain. Never stretch to the point of pain. Static stretching is safest.
- Free weights can be used but machines may be easier to work around limitations.
- Pool exercise can help improve CV endurance.
- When in doubt, increasing time of exercise is safer than the intensity of exercise.
- People with RA tend to have extended joint stiffness in the morning.[176] This may require extra warm up time to compensate.
- Increased pain 1-2 hours after exercise may indicate the person did too much.[176]
- For more information visit the American Arthritis Foundation www.arthritis.org.

Fibromyalgia Syndrome Guidelines

Key Points

- A condition highlighted by widespread pain and stiffness felt in the muscles, ligaments and tendons. Pain is felt at specific areas (tender points) of the body.
- Classified as a type of arthritis. The cause of fibromyalgia is unknown. Some research suggests it may be related to a hypersensitivity of nerves which conduct feelings of pain in response to stimuli that normally isn't painful.
- To be diagnosed: 1.) Must be in pain for at least 3 months and 2.) Pain must be specific to tender points. All other causes of symptoms must be ruled out also.
- Tender points include those of upper chest, back of the head, upper back, neck, elbows, hips and knees. Fatigue and depression are also common as is numbness in hands and/or feet.
- Pain varies according to emotions, stress, exercise, lack of sleep.
- May be sensitive to cold, touch and bright lights. Migraine headaches may also occur.
- People may not sleep well. Lack of quality sleep appears to increase feelings of pain/fatigue.

General Exercise Guidelines

Type of Exercise	Exercise Guideline	Frequency, Intensity, Time
Aerobic	Use large muscle groups	Low intensity. Focus on time of exercise rather than intensity
Strength training	Little research. Use light resistance	Light resistances. Increasing reps performed may be safer than increasing resistances used.
Flexibility	Stretch before exercise, during exercise, after exercise and throughout the day	Stretch to mild discomfort only. Never stretch to pain.

Comments & Suggestions

- Help the person feel better and improve ADLs if needed. Exercise programs should be gentle. Exercise alone will not cure fibromyalgia, but it can help.
- Pain levels can wax and wane, making it difficult to continually ramp up the exercise program. Exercise intensity should not be the main focus of the program.
- Don't exercise to fatigue or muscle failure. This may make symptoms worse.
- Warm water pool exercise may help with pain levels.
- Some may have conditions other than fibromyalgia.
- Some may also have chronic fatigue syndrome which is different than fibromyalgia, however, there are common symptoms between the disorders.
- For more information visit the National Fibromyalgia Association www.fmaware.org.

Osteoporosis Guidelines

Key Points

➢ Defined as brittle bone disorder
➢ Type I osteoporosis occurs between 50-70 yrs of age. Type II after 70 years of age.
➢ Mostly affects postmenopausal women. Usually significant in men after age 70.
➢ Poor/inadequate nutrition can promote osteoporosis at younger ages. By the 40s some bone loss has probably occurred. Building strong bones in youth reduces prevalence in old age.
➢ Osteopenia: significant bone loss but not yet to point of osteoporosis. May progress to osteoporosis unless intervention occurs.
➢ Common bones fractured from falls: hips and wrist bones.
➢ Bone cells: osteoblasts are bone-making cells. Osteocytes are mature bone cells. Osteoclasts are bone-eating cells.
➢ Estrogen causes death to osteoclasts and extends life of osteoblasts. After menopause, estrogen decreases and osteoclast activity ramps up, accelerating bone loss.
➢ Risk factors: gender, ethnicity, genetics, age, thin bones and lifestyle factors.
➢ Life style factors: lack of calcium and vitamin D, lack of exercise, smoking, excess alcohol.

General Exercise Guidelines[141]

Type of Exercise	Exercise Guideline	Frequency, Intensity, Time
Aerobic	Multi-joint activities	40-70% maximum heart rate. 20-30 minutes per session, most days of the week
Strength training	Multi joint activities; machines or free weights, etc appropriate	2-3 sets of 50% 1RM or 70% 3RM, performed for 8 reps. 2 days per week

Comments & Suggestions

➢ If a novice has osteoporosis, start with lighter weights for first few months to let the body adapt before loading it with heavier resistances. This will reduce injury.
➢ Include balance and/or functional training activities to improve hand-eye coordination and ADLs.
➢ Some evidence suggests crunches on the floor may increase fractures of spinal column.
➢ For very deconditioned people, chair-based exercise programs may be needed.
➢ Some people may have conditions other than osteoporosis. The guidelines for these other conditions may clash with guidelines for osteoporosis.
➢ The characteristic curved upper back (hunch back) of many with osteoporosis may reduce the ability to breathe and thus impact exercise.
➢ Calcium supplements: calcium carbonate is cheapest and has most usable calcium per supplement. Calcium RDA: 1200-1500 mg/day.
➢ It may take at least a year before a noticeable impact on bone mass from exercise training is observed.
➢ For more information visit the National Osteoporosis Foundation www.nof.org.

Multiple Sclerosis Guidelines

Key Points

- Myelin is a fatty material that insulates and protects nerves and helps speed the transmission of nerve impulses in the central nervous system (CNS).
- MS results in an erosion (demyelination) of myelin. This causes a reduction in the speed of nerve transmission and a disruption of coordinated movements.
- The muscles of those with MS may contract involuntarily. This is referred to as *muscle spasticity*. This may result in awkward movements during walking and/or exercise. Treadmill exercise may be difficult for this population.
- As body temperature rises, muscle spasticity increases. Thus, frequent rest periods may be needed to maintain optimal body temperature.
- People with MS may also suffer from widespread pain.
- Symptoms can include disruptions to vision as well as problems with bowels, coordination, fatigue and pain.
- Symptoms can be relapsing in nature (coming and going). Most cases are this type. Symptoms may also be progressive, in which case, getting steadily worse overtime.[178]
- Women are twice as likely to get MS than men are.[178]
- MS is thought to result from an autoimmune disorder where the immune system attacks the myelin covering. What causes the immune system to go awry is unknown. While a genetic link may exists, some research hints that exposure to environmental toxins (virus, bacteria, industrial toxin etc.) early in life (before age 15) may predispose the person to MS later on.[179] Those who live in high-risk areas who move to low risk areas before 15 are at lower risk of MS later in life.[179] Some also feel there may be a link to low levels of vitamin D.[179]
- MS can occur at any age but mostly affects people between 15-50 years of age.[178]

General Exercise Guidelines

Type of Exercise	Exercise Guideline	Frequency, Intensity, time
Aerobic	Large muscle groups	3 days per week, ≤ 70% HR max, 30 min per session
Strength Training	Perform on different days than cardio	1-3 sets of 8-15 RM

Symptoms of Multiple Sclerosis*

↓ Coordination	Muscle fatigue	Slurred speech
↓ Attention span	Muscle atrophy	Urinary incontinence
Dizziness/ loss of balance	Muscle spasms	Uncontrolled rapid eye movements

*Partial list

Comments & Suggestions

➤ The goals of exercise are to slow the physical manifestations of MS and maintain and/or improve fitness levels as well as help the person improve ADLs and quality of life.

➤ Exercising the hands/fingers and even making faces can be part of the exercise program.

➤ Depending on fitness levels, starting with low level (e.g., 10 minutes) and gradually increasing time as fitness progresses may be needed. Intermittent exercise may be needed.

➤ Stretching, both passive and partner assisted, can help improve circulation and may help muscle function.

➤ The environment should be free of any obstacles that can cause tripping. Likewise wet floors may result in more falls in those with MS.

➤ Some people with MS may not sweat very much or not at all. This can cause even moderate exercise to ramp up body temperature, which heightens muscle spasticity. If possible, cooler room temperatures (66-70° F) with low humidity may help.

➤ While pool exercise may help, heated pools may exacerbate symptoms. Likewise steam rooms/saunas should be avoided by those with MS.

➤ Some people with MS may be taking prednisone, an anti-inflammatory steroid that causes muscle weakness. It can also cause bone loss, fatigue, weight gain and reduced wound healing. It can also cause extreme fluctuations in mood.[180]

➤ If balance and/or muscle spasticity are an issue, supervise closely during weight bearing activity Non-weight bearing CV activity (e.g., bike) may also help. Supervise when exiting fitness equipment.

➤ Wearing loose/light clothing can help keep the body cool and reduce muscle spasticity. Adequate hydration and weight loss may also help maintain body temperature elevations.

➤ Intense training may increase muscle spasticity.

➤ Symptoms may change daily which may make exercise progressions difficult.

➤ Some may process information slower than usual. It may be necessary to repeat exercise instructions frequently. Positive reinforcement can help with frustration, depression and exercise adherence.

➤ While free weights can be used, because of muscle spasticity and pain, machines may be safer. That being said, other types of exercise equipment may be used.

➤ Avoid exercise to failure or exhaustion. Rest periods between sets of resistance training should be long enough to allow for recovery and help maintain optimal core temperature.

➤ Modify exercise programs according to MS flair ups and/or progression of the syndrome.

➤ Positive reinforcement should be used to foster exercise adherence.

➤ Remind the person to listen to their body for signs of symptoms worsening with exercise.

➤ Reduce/stop exercise during flair ups and resume the program when symptoms subside

➤ For more information see the National Multiple Sclerosis Society at www.nationalmssociety.org

Prepubescent Children Guidelines

Key Points

> - Discuss with parents the goals – sports performance, sports injury reduction, weight loss, exercise instruction, etc. before exercise training occurs.
> - Exercise programs should include all aspects of fitness –muscular and CV endurance, strength and flexibility. Exercise programs should also be fun for the child.
> - Adult exercise guidelines (e.g., 30-60 min CV activity most days of the week) may not be appropriate for kids because of boredom and because aerobic adaptations to CV exercise may be less dramatic than in adults.[165] Games incorporating CV exercise may be better.
> - Prepubescent boys and girls appear to increase strength to equal degrees.[5]
> - Kids as young as 6 years of age have benefited from properly-designed strength training programs.[166] There is no proof that a weight training program that's supervised by qualified instructors, stunts the growth of kids. Damage to growth plates has not been reported.[5] If not properly designed or supervised, injuries to growth plates may occur however.
> - The intensity of the program should not be too much for the child at his/her stage of development.
> - Before puberty, most strength gains are due to neurological changes rather than increased muscle protein synthesis or hypertrophy.

General Exercise Guidelines

Type of Exercise	Exercise Guideline	Frequency, Intensity, time
Aerobic	No official guidelines. Multi joint activities (games, treadmill, walking, jogging).	No official guidelines. Interval training may mimic how kids play in the real world.
Strength training	Multi joint and single joint activities. Machines, free weights, body weight exercises.	Light resistance (12-20 reps) 2-3 days per week.

Comments & Suggestions

> - Consider the maturity level when developing an exercise program. Can they follow directions or work effectively in small groups?
> - Be someone they feel comfortable approaching. Be open to the child's concerns and possible fears about exercise. Always include a 5-10 minute warm up prior to exercise.
> - It's usually not necessary to determine RM values. Focus on exercise technique and form rather than weight lifted. Resistances lifted for 12-15 reps are usually adequate.
> - Exercise should be fun especially for young kids. Games may be preferable for some.
> - Evidence suggests that properly designed resistance training programs can improve bone density, aerobic fitness, lower cholesterol levels, improve skill performance and improve body composistion.[5]

- Kids take longer to sweat and tend to sweat less than adults. As such, kids may be at greater risk of hyperthermia. Overweight kids may be especially prone because of the insulating effect of excess body weight. Remember to take time to hydrate.
- Educate the child that the maximum amount of weight lifted is not important. Focus on long term health benefits. Speaking in language they can understand and using ideas and phrases common to their generation may enhance the child's exercise education and long term adherence to exercise.

Frail and Older Adult Guidelines

Key Points

- Frail is defined as lacking the strength/endurance to perform 2 or more ADLs, or someone who has sarcopenia.
- It's possible to be young and frail. It's possible to be older and not frail.
- Anything that limits mobility can lead to being frail
- Frailty may also result in other issues (diabetes, obesity, etc.)
- Americans are growing older. People over 85 represent the fastest segment of the older adult population. Most people in nursing homes are also over 85. Thus, Americans are living longer but they have problems with independence and quality of life.
- Proper exercise can help slow and sometimes reverse many aspects of the aging process

General Exercise Guidelines

Type of Exercise	Exercise Guideline	Frequency, Intensity, time
Aerobic	Low intensity. Progress as tolerated	5-60 min/day. 3-5 day/week. Low intensity
Strength training	Start with low intensity. Progress as strength improves	20 min per session/ 3 days per week. Intensity level varies between people

Comments & Suggestions

- There is no universal exercise guideline that can be applied to all people who are frail or elderly. The trick is to look at the whole person: their likes dislikes, abilities, health history, ADLs, limitations and goals and find something that works for them.
- Balance may be an issue and something to incorporate into the exercise program.
- Reducing the risk of falling through exercise and proper movement mechanics can help improve the quality and quantity of life.
- With older individuals, longer rest periods (e.g., 2-5 min) may be needed between sets.
- For older individuals or those using medications that lower HR, the Talk Test and/or Borg scale are preferable to HR when estimating exercise intensity.
- Don't worry about target heart rate in older individuals.
- For those with blood pressure issues, avoid static and isometric exercises.
- Avoid ballistic movements as they may increase injury.
- Functional training may, in some instances, help improve ADLs.
- Because of sarcopenia, frail people will move slower and take longer to react due to reductions in type II fiber density. If possible, targeting type II fibers may improve life quality.
- Frail/older individuals may not consume adequate or quality calories or enough fluids.
- Older adults may have a reduced sensation of thirst, which may lead to dehydration, overheating and reduced exercise capacity. They may also eat less calories and protein and may be less efficient at producing muscle protein.
- Healthy older adults with no medical issues are able to lift heavy weights.[77], Varying the resistance lifted seems to improve strength more than constantly lifting heavy weights.[77]
- Because of weakened condition, exercising to exhaustion is not recommended.

Pregnancy Guidelines

Key Points

- Moderate exercise is safe for women with uncomplicated pregnancy.[167] One of the main goals of the exercise program is to prepare women for the demands of labor and childbirth.
- Sedentary women who start an exercise program while pregnant, must obtain physician's permission first.[1] Progress slowly and within comfort level.[167]
- Women who exercise during pregnancy experience less low back pain compared to sedentary women.[168]
- Fetal size does not appear to be affected by moderate exercise training during pregnancy.[167] Intense exercise (1-2.5 hr/day) may result in lower fat mass of babies.[169]
- Gestational diabetes may occur as a result of increased blood sugar during pregnancy.

Absolute Contraindications to Exercise While Pregnant[167,174]

Pregnant with 3 or more babies (e.g., ≥ triplets)	Pregnancy-induced high blood pressure
Preeclampsia/eclampsia	Bleeding in the 2nd or 3rd trimester
Weak cervix	Women at risk of premature labor
Smoking /alcohol abuse	Previous spontaneous abortion

Possible Contraindications to Exercise that Require Physician's Approval[167,174]

Any cardiovascular problems	Mother is underweight or has eating disorder
Low fitness level	Anemia
Type I or II diabetes	Any significant medical issues

General Exercise Guidelines[167,174]

Type of Exercise	Exercise Guideline	Frequency, Intensity, time
Aerobic	Low intensity	If sedentary, start with 15 min 3 d/wk. Progress to 30 min, 4d/wk. Work until fatigue, never exhaustion.
Strength Training	Train for muscle endurance	Light weight. Increase reps/sets as tolerated.

Comments & Suggestions

- Goals for exercise should be to train for muscle endurance, focusing on muscles involved in labor: maintain ADLs, improve posture during pregnancy, reduce low back pain and strengthen weight bearing muscles.[173]
- Do not exercise to failure or exhaustion. Cease exercise when fatigued.[1]

➢ Machines may, in some instances, be safer than free weights. Pregnancy may preclude the use of some machines because of increased abdominal girth and/or restricted ROM.

➢ Avoid crunches after the 1ˢᵗ trimester. Crunches may cause diastasis — tearing of the rectus abdominis muscle.

➢ After the first trimester, avoid exercises that place the women in the supine (lying on the back) position as this can reduce blood pressure and cardiac output and blood flow to the baby.

➢ Water-based exercise is usually appropriate for this population and helps reduce maternal core temperature and edema and facilitates blood flow to the baby. Scuba diving however should be avoided throughout the pregnancy.

➢ Sedentary women who start an exercise program while pregnant may be at greater risk of medical issues than those who are regular exercisers.

➢ Avoid ballistic–type exercises and those that require excessive balance with added resistances (e.g., lunges, squats, stiff-leg dead lifts).

➢ Avoid activities that require long periods of motionless standing.

➢ Balance issues may arise because of distended abdominal girth. Avoid activities that require fast changes in direction.

➢ Because of hormonal fluctuations (i.e., relaxin), joints may become hyper flexible (laxity) resulting in increased risk of injury.

➢ As pregnancy progresses, less exercise may be able to be performed. Adjust exercise accordingly.

➢ Excessive low back inward curvature (lordosis) may result in back pain. Excessive curvature of the upper back (kyphosis) may cause a rounding of the shoulders.

➢ RHR may rise by 10-15 bpm when pregnant.

➢ Both the talk test and Borg scale can be used to monitor exercise exertion during pregnancy.[167]

➢ Total blood volume may increase in pregnant women by as much as 40% above normal. This could lead to swelling in the arms/legs, nose and gum bleeding, varicose veins and headaches.

➢ At least 300 extra calories per day may be needed during pregnancy because of increased metabolic rate. Women who exercise may need extra calories.[167]

➢ Exercise in hot and/or humid environments is not recommended as it may elevate temperature. This effect may be more pronounced in untrained women.[170]

➢ Maintain adequate hydration. This can help maintain proper core temperature.

➢ Pain in the groin or anterior thigh could, in theory, indicate osteoporosis of the hip.[171] Consult physician for diagnosis.

➢ Fitness testing is not necessary for pregnant women.[174]

➢ Physician approval to exercise may be withdrawn if medical issues arise during pregnancy.

➢ After delivery, exercise should be resumed gradually. At least 6 weeks may be needed before the woman's body returns to the pre-pregnancy state.[1]

Reasons for Stopping Exercise and Seeking Immediate Medical Attention[1]

Fluid discharge from vagina	Unknown loss of consciousness or fainting	Chest pain, rapid HR, fatigue or unknown abdominal pain
Bloody discharge from vagina	Persistent increase in BP or HR after exercise stops	Uterine contractions
Severe headache, vision disruption	Swelling/pain/redness in one calf	Abrupt swelling of ankles, face or hands

Visual Impairments Guidelines

Key Points

➤ Deficits in vision can be caused by a number of factors ranging from cataracts, glaucoma, age-related macular degeneration (AMD) and head trauma to name a few.

General Exercise Guidelines

Type of Exercise	Exercise Guideline	Frequency, Intensity, time
Aerobic	No official guidelines. Large muscle groups	20-60 minutes, most days of the week
Strength Training	No official guidelines	2-3 days per week, intensity and time vary as tolerated according to fitness level

Comments & Suggestions

➤ If visual impairment is the only health issue to consider, these people are considered apparently healthy and can be trained similarly to healthy, sighted individuals with few restrictions. If other issues exist, work within established guidelines for those conditions.

➤ Those with vision issues will likely also have balance detriments. The trainer should stay with the individual and, if needed, physically guide him/her through the workout.

➤ People with vision impairments may have low CV endurance and strength due to reduced ability to exercise alone. This may lead to various associated conditions such as weight gain and type II diabetes. Heart disease is possible also.

➤ Individuals may suffer from a fear/anxiety of unfamiliar surroundings (e.g., gym). Trainers should be aware of this and work to foster a bond of trust with the person.

➤ Verbal and physical cues/instructions are especially important if using free weights. The trainer should help the lifter with the lift-off and re-racking of the weight.

➤ If blindness was caused by physical trauma (detached retina) or he/she recently had cataract surgery, avoid activities that are high impact.[141] Likewise, heavy weightlifting/intense cardio is not advised after recent eye surgery. Facial deformity may also be present following physical trauma which may further foster feelings of anxiety on the part of the individual.

➤ If exercising in a health club, the trainer should walk the person around the facility to make them aware of landmarks, emergency exits, stairs, locker rooms and other important features.

➤ If working out in a pool, the facility should place an audible sound (e.g., radio) at the shallow end of the pool to help the person differentiate the deep and shallow ends.

➤ Exercise should stop and the person referred to their eye doctor if any worsening of vision occurs during exercise.

Glossary

Abduction. To move a body part away from the body. Sometimes called Ab-duction.

Actin. A muscle protein. One of the myofilaments found in myofibrils.

Acute. In exercise, usually refers to a short-term change. *Chronic* refers to long term change.

Adduction. To move a body part closer to the body: Sometimes called AD-duction..

ADL. Activity of daily living. Tasks performed on a regular basis. Walking, going to the bathroom are ADLs. IADLs are instrumental activities of daily living. IADLs refer to paying bills, cooking, laundry and shopping.

Aerobic Exercise. Exercise that uses oxygen to generate energy (ATP). Also called cardiovascular exercise.

Anaerobic Exercise. Exercise that does not require oxygen to make energy (ATP).

Antagonist Muscle. The muscle or muscles which oppose the prime mover. Antagonists help slow down joint movement and overall help reduce joint injury. *See also prime mover.*

Articular cartilage. Joint cartilage found at the ends of bones.

ATP. Adenosine Triphosphate. The body's ultimate energy molecule.

bpm. Abbreviation for beats per minute.

BMD. Bone mineral density. Osteoporosis results in a reduction in BMD

BMI. Body mass index.

BMR. Basal Metabolic Rate. The lowest metabolism possible. *See also RMR.*

Body Composition. The amount of fat and fat-free mass that a body contains.

Borg Scale. A 0-10 scale used to estimate exercise intensity. Also called RPE scale.

Carbohydrate. Carbohydrates are sugars. The main energy source used during exercise.

Cardiovascular Exercise. Aerobic exercise.

Closed Grip. In weight lifting, a closed grip occurs when the thumbs are wrapped around the bar of the free weight or handle of weight machine.

Concentric Muscle Action. In weightlifting, the phase of a muscle contraction where the weight is lifted. Also called "positives". *See also eccentric.*

Core. In exercise, all the muscles of the trunk.

CNS. Central nervous system. Consists of the brain and spinal cord.

COPD. Chronic Obstructive Pulmonary Disorder. Lung disease that makes it hard to breath like emphysema or chronic bronchitis. COPD is the 4th leading cause of death. Smoking is the primary risk factor for COPD.

CPT. Certified Personal Trainer.

Creatine Phosphate. An energy source that helps regenerate ATP during periods of intense physical activity.

CRP. C-Reactive Protein. Elevations of CRP may be linked to heart disease.

DOMS. Delayed Onset Muscle Soreness.

Diastolic Blood Pressure. The pressure of the blood on the walls of the blood vessels when the heart is in its filling phase. *See also systolic BP and blood pressure*

Eccentric Muscle Action. In weightlifting, the phase of a muscle contraction where the weight is lowered. Also called "negatives". *See also concentric.*

Ejection Fraction. The percentage of blood pumped from the heart with each heart beat.

Electrolytes. Elements that allow electrical impulses to be transmitted in biological systems. Sodium, potassium, calcium and chloride are examples of electrolytes.

EPOC. Excessive Post-exercise Oxygen Consumption. EPOC refers to the elevation in metabolism that occurs after exercise. The older name is oxygen debt. *See also NEAT.*

Fast twitch muscle. Type II muscle fiber.

FITT Principle. Frequency, Intensity, Time and Type of exercise.

Free Weight. Barbells and dumbbells.

Gluconeogenesis. The making of sugar (glucose) from non carbohydrate substances (e.g. protein).

Glucose. Blood sugar. Normal blood sugar is less than 100 mg/dl.

Glycogen. Storage form of glucose.

Glycolysis. The chemical pathway responsible for the breakdown of sugar (glucose) for energy (ATP) that does not require oxygen. Glycolysis is an anaerobic energy system.

Gram. Unit of weight in the metric system. There are 28 grams in one ounce.

HDL. High density lipoprotein. The so-called "good" cholesterol. *See also LDL and cholesterol.*

Hemoglobin A1c. A marker of long term blood sugar levels (~3 months). Elevated levels increase risk of heart disease. Also abbreviated as HbA1c.

Homeostasis. Refers to maintaining an internal balance. Our ability to survive as our environment changes is ultimately due to our body's ability to keep the status quo.

HR. abbreviation for Heart Rate. Maximum heart rate is abbreviated as Max HR or HRmax

Hyperplasia. Refers to an increase in cell number. See also hypertrophy.

Hypertension. High blood pressure. Abbreviated as HTN.

Hypertrophy. An increase in size. *See also hyperplasia.*

Hypoglycemia. Low blood sugar levels.

Idiopathic. A condition that has no known cause.

Isometric Muscle Action. A type of muscle action in which the muscle does not change in length while force is applied to it. Also called static contractions.

Isotonic Muscle Action. A type of muscle action where the tension on the muscle remains constant while the muscle changes its length. Composed to two phases called concentric and eccentric.

Kilogram. One kilogram = 1,000 grams. One kilogram (1 kg) is equal to about 2.2 pounds.

Krebs Cycle. The chemical reaction series that involves the aerobic breakdown of fat.

Lactate. A metabolic byproduct of glycolysis made during the anaerobic breaking down sugar (glucose) for energy (ATP). Production coincides with burning sensation during felt during intense exercise. Sometimes called lactic acid.

LDL. Low density lipoprotein. The so-called "bad" cholesterol.

Macronutrient. Nutrients that make up the greatest amount of our diet. Proteins, fats and carbohydrates are the macronutrients.

MET. Metabolic equivalents. 1 MET is equal to 3.5 milliliters of oxygen per kilogram of body weight per minute. METs are another way to measure exercise intensity.

Metabolic Syndrome. Several symptoms that tend to occur together that appear to increase risk of type II diabetes. Used to be called syndrome X. *See also CRP.*

Metabolism. The total of all the chemical reactions (anabolic + catabolic) in the body. Also, the speed at which we burn calories.

M.I. Abbreviation for myocardial infarction. A heart attack.

Mitochondria. A region of the cell where fat is broken down to generate energy (ATP).

Multi Joint Exercise. A movement that uses many muscles simultaneously. Also called a compound exercise. Example. Leg press. *See also single joint exercise.*

Myofibril. Basically, complexes of myosin and actin proteins (and other proteins) that make up muscle fibers.

Myoglobin. An oxygen-carrying compound in muscle cells that's similar to hemoglobin.

Myosin. A muscle protein. One of the myofilaments found in myofibrils.

NEAT. non-exercise activity thermogenesis. Basically any activity, other than exercise, that burns calories. Examples: shopping, gardening, working. May play a role in weight loss and weight maintenance. *See also EPOC.*

Neutral grip. In weight lifting, when the hands are facing each other

Obese. Excessively overweight. A BMI greater than 30 is considered obese.

Osteoporosis. A disease where bones become brittle and break easily. Osteoporosis effects both men and women.

OT. Occupational Therapist. *See also PT*

Overtraining Syndrome. A phenomenon that occurs when people regularly exercise to exhaustion and don't get enough rest between exercise sessions.

Oxygen Consumption. The amount of oxygen that can be used to make energy aerobically. Higher consumptions are associated with greater aerobic fitness.

Periodization. An exercise protocol in which an exercise program is divided into different cycles or phases. Different goals are addressed in each of the various periodization phases. The main objectives of periodization are to maximize training goals while reducing injury.

Power. Power is explosive strength. Power does not last long (e.g. 20-30 seconds). Strength and power are not the same. Strength generally lasts for 2-5 minutes.

Preeclampsia. High blood pressure occurring during pregnancy and post-pregnancy. Eclampsia refers to seizures during pregnancy.

Prehypertension. A consistent, resting blood pressure that's 120/80 mm Hg – 139/89 mm Hg.

Prime Mover. The muscle primary responsible for the movement. Also called the agonist.

Prone. Anatomical position where the person is laying on his/her stomach. The pronated position also when the palms of the hands are facing downward. *See also supine.*

Protein. One of the macronutrients. Proteins are made of smaller units called amino acids.

PT. Physical Therapist. *See also OT.*

RD. Registered Dietitian.

Repetition. One complete cycle of an exercise. Example, lifting a weight 12 times means you performed 12 repetitions. Abbreviated as "rep". *See also set.*

RHR. Resting heart rate.

RM. Repetition Maximum. The most weight one can lift for a certain number of times with good lifting technique.

RMR. Resting Metabolic Rate.

RPE Scale. Ratings of Perceived Exertion Scale. The Borg Scale.

Sarcomere. The basic unit of muscle contraction.

Sarcopenia. Loss of muscle as we grow older.

Sedentary. One who does not exercise regularly.

Selectorized Machine. Type of strength training machine where the resistance can be selected (e.g. inserting a pin into a weight stack).

Set. A group of repetitions (reps).

Single-Joint Exercise. An exercise that uses smaller amounts of muscles.

Skeletal muscle. Muscles that are attached to the skeleton. Biceps for example.

Slow twitch muscle. Type I muscle fibers

Soft-Lock Out. A soft lock out occurs when the joint is not totally locked out.

Special Populations. Phrase used for anyone who has a special need. Examples include those with osteoporosis, high blood pressure or heart disease.

Spotting. A spotter is a lifting partner (or trainer) who spots and corrects errors in exercise technique and/or assists the lifter performing the movement.

Sticking Point. The most difficult part of a weight lifting movement.

Supine. Anatomical position when one is lying on the back. Supination also occurs when the palms of the hands are facing upward. *See also prone.*

Synergist Muscle. A helper muscle. A synergist muscle acts in synergy or cooperation with the prime mover to accomplish the task at hand. *See also prime mover.*

Systolic Blood Pressure. The pressure of the blood on the walls of the blood vessels when the heart is in its contraction phase.

THR. Target Heart Rate.

Triglyceride. Another name for fat. Triglycerides are stored in fat cells and are released into the blood when needed such as during exercise.

Type I Muscle Fibers. Slow twitch fibers.

Type II Muscle Fibers. Fast twitch fibers.

Valsalva Maneuver. Holding one's breath during exercise.

VO$_2$ The volume of oxygen used to make energy aerobically. Used as a measure of exercise intensity and aerobic fitness. *See also oxygen consumption and METs.*

Volume. In exercise, defined as the weight x reps x sets. Example, performing 2 sets of an exercise at 100 lbs for 10 reps is 100 X 10 X 2 = 2000 lbs.

Sample Health History Form

Today's Date _____

Name _____

Address _____

City / State / Zip _____

Phone (H) _____

Phone (W) _____

Primary Email _____

Date of Birth _____

Age _____

Weight (lb.) _____   Height (in) _____

Emergency Contact Information

Name _____   Relationship _____

Phone (H)_____   Phone (W) _____

Name of Personal Physician

Dr. Name _____

Office address _____

Office Telephone _____

Personal Health History

Do you now have or have you had in the past, any of the following conditions or syndromes?

1. Heart attack   yes   no
2. Chest pain at rest   yes   no
3. Chest pain during physical activity   yes   no
4. Heart surgery   yes   no
5. Irregular heart beat   yes   no
6. Do you have a pacemaker   yes   no
7. Other heart problems not listed above   yes   no

8. If yes, please explain _____

_____

9. High cholesterol   yes   no
10. High triglycerides   yes   no
11. Stroke   yes   no
12. Diabetes   yes   no
13. If yes, what type do you have: Type I   Type II
14. Osteoarthritis   yes   no

15. Rheumatoid arthritis	yes	no
16. Asthma	yes	no
17. Emphysema	yes	no

18. Currently pregnant   yes   no

19. Cancer	yes	no
20. Recent surgery	yes	no
21. History of neck problems	yes	no
22. History of back problems	yes	no
23. History of knee problems	yes	no
24. History of shoulder problems	yes	no
25. Hearing problems	yes	no
26. Vision problems	yes	no
27. Problems maintaining balance	yes	no
28. Osteoporosis	yes	no
29. High blood pressure	yes	no
30. Other medical problems not listed above	yes	no

31. If yes, please explain _____

32. When was your last physical? _____

33. Do you currently smoke?   yes   no

34. Do you ever experience spells of severe dizziness? yes   no

35. Have you undergone physical therapy in the last 2 years? _____

36. Do you ever experience shortness of breath? _____

37. Do you have any other health issue not mentioned above? _____

_____

Family Medical History

Do you have a family history of any of the following?

Diabetes	yes	no
Cancer	yes	no
Osteoporosis	yes	no
Heart disease	yes	no
Stroke	yes	no
Obesity	yes	no

Are both parents still alive?   yes   no

If not, how old were they and what was the cause of death? _____

_____

Medications

To the best of your knowledge, please list all medications you are taking and the reasons you are taking them _____

_____

_____

References

1. ACSM's Guidelines for Exercise Testing and Prescription, 6th edition. Lippincott Williams & Williams.

2. Heyward, VH (1991). Advanced Fitness Assessment & Exercise Prescription. Second edition. Human Kinetics.

3. Heyward, VH (1997). Advanced Fitness Assessment & Exercise Prescription. Third edition. Human Kinetics.

4. Golding LA, Myers CA and Sinning WE (1989). Y's Way to Physical Fitness, 3rd edt. Human Kinetics.

5. Earl RW & Baechle TR (2004). NSCA's Essentials of Personal Training. Human Kinetics.

6. No authors. One Rep Maximum. wikipedia.org/wiki/One_rep_maximum (accessed 11/26/06).

7. No authors. Department of Health and Human Services. www.surgeongeneral.gov/topics/obesity/calltoaction/fact_consequences.htm (accessed 12/5/06).

8. McArdle, W. D., Katch, F. I., Katch, V. L. (1999). Sport & Exercise Nutrition. Lippincott, Williams & Wilkins.

9. Broeder CE (1997). Assessing body composition before and after resistance or endurance training. Medicine and Science in Sports and Exercise, 29,5, 705-712.

10. Maddalozzo, G. F..et al. (2002). Concurrent validity of the BOD POD and dual nergy x-ray absorptiometry techniques for assessing body composition in young women. Journal of the American Dietetic Association, 102,11,1677 1679.

11. Utter, A.C. et al. (2003). Evaluation of air displacement for assessing body composition of collegiate wrestlers. Medicine and Science in Sports and Exercise, 35,3, 00-505.

12. Vescovi, J. D. et al. (2002). Evaluation of the BOD POD for estimating percent fat in female college athletes. Journal of Strength and Conditioning Research, 16, 4, 599-605.

13. Vescovi, J.D. et al. (2001). Evaluation of the BOD POD for estimating percentage body fat in a heterogeneous group of adult humans. European Journal of Applied Physiology, 85, 3-4, 326-332.

14. Lockner D.W. et al. (2000). Comparison of air-displacement plethysmography, hydrodensitometry, and dual X-ray absorptiometry for assessing body composition of children 10 to 18 years of age. Annals of the New York Academy of Science, 904, 72-78.

15. Jouven X et al (2005).Heart rate profile during exercise as a predictor of sudden death. New England Journal of Medicine, 12,352 (19), 1951-1958.

16. Brooks D (1997). Program Design for Personal Trainers. Moves International.

17. Chobanian AV et al (2003). The seventh report of the joint national committee on prevention, detection, evaluation and treatment of high blood pressure. The JNC 7 report. JAMA, 289,19,2560-2572.

18. No author. Heart. How It Works. American Heart Association. www.americanheart.org/presenter.jhtml?identifier=4642 (accessed 1/8/07)

19. MacReady, N. Drugs and Athletes: It's All About the Gold. www.webmd.com/content/article/36/1728_61278.htm (accessed 1/12/07)

20. Maltin LJ (2001). Share and Share Alike – Except in the Locker Room. www.webmd.com/content/article/36/1676_52814.htm (accessed 1/16/07).

21. Rhoades RA, Tanner GA (editors) (2003). *Medical Physiology*, 2nd ed., Lippincott Williams & Wilkins.

22. Stryer, L (1988). Biochemistry, 3rd edt W.H. Freeman and Company.

23. No author. An Introduction to Carbon Monoxide. Environmental Protection Agency. www.epa.gov/iaq/co.html#Health%20Effects%20Associated%20with%20Carbon%20Monoxide (accessed 1/16/07).

24. Guyton AC et al. (1996). Textbook of Medical Physiology, 9th edition.

25. Howley ET and Franks BD (1997). Health Fitness Instructor's Handbook. 3rd edition. Human Kinetics.

26. Persinger R et al (2004). Consistency of the talk test for exercise prescription. Medicine and Science in Sports and Exercise, 36,9, 1632-1636.

27. Rubal BJ et al (1987). Effects of physical conditioning on the heart size and wall thickness of college women. Medicine and Science in Sports and Exercise 19,5,423-429

28. Kiens B et al (1993). Skeletal muscle substrate utilization during submaximal exercise in man.: Effects of endurance training. Journal of Physiology, 469,459-478.

29. Powers SK and Howley ET (1990). Exercise Physiology: Theory and Application to Fitness and Performance. Second edition. Brown & Benchmark.

30. Fox E, Bowers R and Foss M (1993). The Physiological Basis for Exercise and Sport. Fifth edition. Brown & Benchmark.

31. Sugiura H et al (2002). Effects of long term moderate exercise and increase in number of daily steps on serum lipids in women. Randomized control trial. BMC Women's Health, 2:3 www.biomedcentral.com/1472-6874/2/3 (accessed 2/13/07).

32. Pate, RR., et al (1995). Physical activity and public health: A recommendation from the Centers for Disease Control and Prevention and the American College of Sports Medicine. *JAMA*. 273:402–407. 1995.

33. Quinn TJ et al. (2006). Two short daily activity bouts vs. one long bout: are health and fitness improvements similar over twelve and twenty-four weeks? Journal of Strength and Conditioning Research, 20,1, 130-135.

34. Adams AK et al. (2002). The role of antioxidants in exercise and disease prevention. Physician and Sports Medicine, 30,5 www.physsportsmed.com/issues/2002/05_02/adams.htm (accessed 2/13/07).

35. No authors. General physical activities defined by level of intensity. Center for Disease Control and Prevention. www.cdc.gov/nccdphp/dnpa/physical/pdf/PA_Intensity_table_2_1.pdf (accessed 2/14/07).

36. Ainsworth BE. (2002, January) The Compendium of Physical Activities Tracking Guide. Prevention Research Center, Norman J. Arnold School of Public Health, University of South Carolina. http://prevention.sph.sc.edu/tools/compendium.htm (accessed 2/14/07).

37. Maxwell AJ et al. (2002). Randomized trial of a medical food for the dietary management of chronic, stable angina. Jouirnal of the American College of Cardiology, 39, 37-45.

38. Cannon, J (2006). Nutritional Supplements: What Works and Why. A Review from A to Zinc and Beyond. Available at www.joe-cannon.com.

39. Nieman, DC (1998). The Exercise-Health Connection. Human Kinetics.

40. US Bureau of Labor and Statistics. www.ubs.gov (accessed Jan 5 2007).

41. Cerny FT and Burton HW (2001). Exercise Physiology for Health Car Professionals. Human Kinetics.

42. Wilmore JH & Costill DL ((1994). Physiology of Sport and Exercise. Human Kinetics.

43. Physical Activity and Health. Chapter 3: Physiologic Responses and Long-Term Adaptations to Exercise. Center for Disease Control and Prevention. www.cdc.gov/nccdphp/sgr/chap3.htm (accessed 2/22/07).

44. Peters, R.K., Bateman, E.D. (1983). Ultramarathon running an upper respiratory track infections. South_African Medical Journal, 64, 582-584.

45. Kohut M, et al. (2002). Exercise and psychosocial factors modulate immunity to influenza vaccine in elderly individuals. Journal of Gerontology, 57A(9): M557–M562.

46. Fiscella, C. (2005). The Lumbar Spine. IDEA Fitness Journal. May, 34-37.

47. No authors. Your high blood pressure questions answered – blood pressure and exercise. American Heart Association www.americanheart.org/presenter.jhtml?identifier=3034814 (accessed 3/8/07).

48. Newham, et al. (1987). Repeated high - Force Eccentric Exercise: Effects on Muscle Pain and Damage. Journal of Applied Physiology 63,41381-1386.

49. Margetic S et al. (2002). Leptin: a review of its peripheral actions and interactions. International Journal of Obesity 26 1407–1433.

50. Kojima, M. et. al. (1999). Ghrelin is a growth hormone releasing acylated peptide from stomach. Nature, 402, 656-660.

51. Finn DA et al. (2005). A new look at the 5-alpha-reductase inhibitor finesteride. CNS Drug Reviews,12,1,53-76.

52. Komi PV (1992). Strength and Power in Sport. Blackwell.

53. Ricoy, J.R., A.R. Encinas, A. Cabello, S. Madero, and J. Arenas. Histochemical study of the vastus lateralis muscle fibre types of athletes. *J. Physiol. Biochem.* 54(1):41-47. 1998.

54. Staron RS et al. (2000). Fiber type composition of the vastus lateralis of young men and women. Journal of Histochemistry and Cytochemistry, 48, 623-630.

55.Suter E et al. (1993). Muscle fiber type distribution as estimated by Cybex testing and by muscle biopsy. Medicine and Science in Sport and Exercise 25,3, 363-370.

56. Douris PC et al. (2006). The relationship between maximal repetition performance and muscle fiber type as estimated by non-invasive technique of quadriceps of untrained women. Journal of Strength and Conditioning, 20,3,699-703.

57. Karp J . Designing programs that work best for your clients. Fitness Management www.fitnessmanagement.com/FM/tmpl/genPage.asp?p=/information/articles/library/features/0601features2.html (accessed 7/29/07).

58. Jannson E et al. (1990). Increase in the proportion of type II muscle fibers by sprint training in males. Acta Physiol Scand. 140,3,359-63.

59. Alway, S. E., P. K. et al. (1989). Regionalized adaptations and muscle fiber proliferation in stretch-induced enlargement. Journal of Applied Physiology, 66,2, 771-781.

60. Yamada, S., N. et. al. (1989). Fibroblast growth factor is stored in fiber extracellular matrix and plays a role in regulating muscle hypertrophy. Medicine and Science in Sports and Exercise. 21,5, S173-S180.

61. Schantz, P et al. (1981). The relationship between mean muscle fiber area and the muscle cross-sectional area of the thigh in subjects with large differences in thigh girth. Acta Physiol. Scand. 113: 537-539.

62. Brown LE (2007). Strength Training. National Strength & Conditioning Association. Human Kinetics.

63. Doherty T (2003). Invited interview: sarcopenia and aging. Journal of Applied Physiology, 95,1717-1727.

64. Baumgartner, RN et al. (1998). Epidemiology of sarcopenia among the elderly in New Mexico. American Journal of Epidemiology, 147,8, 755–763.

65. Greenlund, LJS et al. (2003). Sarcopenia—Consequences, mechanisms, and potential therapies. Mechanisms of Aging and Development, 124,287–299.

66. Bortz, W.M. (2001). Nonage vs. age. Journal of Gerontology: Medical Sciences 56(9): M527-M528.

67. Brooks C. Understanding sarcopenia. Fitness Management. www.fitnessmanagement.com/FM/information/articles/0906-feature3.html (accessed 8/18/07).

68. Sreekumaran K (2004). What is sarcopenia? Mayo Clinic. www.medicaledge.org/newspaper/n-2004october24.html (accessed 8/019/07).

69. Wilderson J (2004). Sarcopenia and exercise: Mechanisms, interactions and application of research findings. Strength and Conditioning Journal, 26,6, 26-31.

70. Balagopal P et al. (1997). Effects of aging on in vivo synthesis of skeletal muscle myosin heavy-chain and sarcoplasmic protein in humans. American Journal of Physiology, 273:E790–E800.

71. Schulte JN et al. (2001). Effects of resistance training on the rate of muscle protein synthesis in frail elderly people. International Journal of Sport Nutrition and Exercise Metabolism, 11:S111–S118.

72. Cannon Joe (2006). Nutritional Supplements: What Works and Why. A Review from A to Zinc –And Beyond. Available at www.Joe-Cannon.com.

73. Yarasheski KE et al. (1999). Resistance exercise training increases mixed muscle proteins synthesis in frail men and women ≥76 years old. American Journal of Physiology Endocrinology and Metabolism, 277: E118-E125.

74. Pichon C et al. (1996). Blood pressure and heart rate and metabolic cost of circuit vs. traditional weight training. Journal of Strength and Conditioning 10,3,135-156.

75. No author. What are high blood pressure and prehypertension? National Heart Lung Blood Institute. http://www.nhlbi.nih.gov/hbp/hbp/whathbp.htm (accessed 8/21/07).

76. Fleck SJ et al. (1997). Designing Resistance Training Programs, 2nd edt. Human Kinetics.

77. Fleck SJ et al. (2003). Designing Resistance Training Programs, 3rd edition. Human Kinetics.

78. Bachle TR and Earle RW (2000). Essentials of Strength Training and Conditioning, 2nd edt. Human Kinetics.

79. Drummond, MJ et al. (2005). Aerobic and resistance exercise sequence affects excess postexercise oxygen consumption. Journal of Strength and Conditioning Research, 19,2,332-337.

80. Hultman E et al. (1996). Muscle creatine loading in men. Journal of Applied Physiology 81,1,232-237.

81. Vandenberghe K et al. (1996). Caffeine counteracts the ergogenic action of muscle creatine loading. Journal of Applied Physiology, 80,452-457.

82. Hespel P (2002). Opposite actions of caffeine and creatine on muscle relaxation time in humans. Journal of Applied Physiology, 92, 512-518.

83. Mayhew D (2002). Effects of long term creatine supplementation on liver and kidney function in American college football players. International Journal of Sports Nutrition and Exercise Metabolism, 12,453-460.

84. Brosnan JT et al. (2007). Creatine: endogenous metabolite, dietary and therapeutic supplement. Annual Review of Nutrition, 27,241-261.

85. Joubert LM et al. (2006). Exercise, nutrition and homocysteine. International Journal of Sports Nutrition and Exercise Metabolism, 16,341-361.

86. McArdle, W. D., Katch, F. I., Katch, V. L. (1999). Sport & Exercise Nutrition. Lippincott, Williams & Wilkins.

87. Press release May 23 2006. Curves. New study shows curves workout can burn more than 500 calories in 30 minutes.

88. Staron RS (1991). Strength and skeletal muscle adaptations in heavy resistance trained women after detaining and retraining. Journal of Applied Physiology, 70,631-640.

89. No author. Heart attack, stroke and cardiac arrest warning signs. www.americanheart.org (accessed 9/24/07).

90. Vingren J and Krarmer WJ (2006). Effect of postexercise alcohol consumption on serum testosterone. A brief review of testosterone, resistance exercise and alcohol. Strength and Conditioning Journal, 28,1,84-87.

91. Schwab, R. et. al. (1993). Acute effects of different intensities of weight lifting on serum testosterone. Medicine and Science in Sports and Exercise, 25,12, 1381-1385.

92. Hakkien K et al. (1988). Neuromuscular and hormonal adaptations in athletes to strength training in two years. Journal of Applied Physiology, 65,2406-2412.

93. Jensen J, et al. (1991). Comparison of changes in testosterone concentrations after strength and endurance exercise in well trained men. European Journal of Applied Physiology, 63, 467-471.

94. Dressendorfer RH et al. (1991). Effects of a 15-d race on plasma steroid levels and leg muscle fitness in runners. Medicine and Science in Sports and Exercise, 23, 954-958.

95. Stone M et al. (1995). Human growth hormone: physiological functions and ergogenic efficiency, Strength and Conditioning, August, pp. 72-74.

96. Rudman D et al. (1990). Effects of human growth hormone in men over 60 years of age. New England Journal of Medicine, 323,1-6.

97. Haff GG (2006). Roundtable discussion: anabolic androgenic steroids part 1. Strength and Conditioning Journal, 28,6,42-55.

98. Kadi F (2000). Adaptations of human skeletal muscle to training and anabolic steroids. Acta Physiologica, 646 (suppl) 1-52.

99. Hickson R et al. (1990). Glucocorticoid antagonism by exercise and anabolic androgenic steroids. Medicine and Science in Sports and Exercise, 22,331-340.

100. Evans, N (2004). Current concepts in anabolic-androgenic steroids. American Journal of Sports Medicine, 32,2,534-542.

101. Parssien M et al. (2002). Steroid use and long term health risks. International Journal of Sports Medicine, 23,83-94.

102. Kraemer WJ et al .(1996). The effects of plasma cortisol evaluation on total and differential leukocyte counts in response to heavy resistance exercise. European Journal of Applied Physiology 73, 1-2, 93-97.

103. Anderson JC (2005). Stretching before and after exercise: effect on muscle soreness and injury risk. Journal of Athletic Training, 40,3 218–220.

104. Shrier, I (2005). When and whom to stretch. Gauging the Benefits and Drawbacks for Individual Patients. Physician and Sports Medicine, 33-3 www.physsportsmed.com/issues/2005/0305/shrier.htm (accessed 2/23/07).

105. Pope HG et al. (1990). Homicide and near-homicide symptoms associated with anabolic steroid use. American Journal of Psychiatry, 145, 487-490.

106. Wright KCS et al. (2002). Infant acceptance of breast milk after maternal exercise. Pediatrics 109,4, 585-589.

107. Graves JE et al. (1988). Effects of reduced training frequency on muscular strength. International Journal of Sports Medicine 9,316-319.

108. Staron, R.S., et al. (1994). Skeletal muscle adaptations during early phase of heavy-resistance training in men and women. Journal of Applied Physiology. 76,1247–1255.

109. Hakkinen, K. et al. (1988). Neuromuscular and hormonal adaptations in athletes to strength training in two years. Journal of Applied Physiology, 65, 2406–2412.

110. MacDougall, JD (1995). The time course for elevated muscle protein synthesis following heavy resistance exercise. Canadian Journal of Applied Physiology, 20,480–486.

111. Burger ME and Burger TA (2002). Neuromuscular and hormonal adaptations to resistance training: Implications for strength development in female athletes. Strength and Conditioning Journal, 24,3, 51-59.

112. Baechle TR & Earle RW (2000). Essentials of Strength and Conditioning, 2nd edt. Human Kinetics.

113. Kleiner S (2007). Power Eating, 3rd edition. Human Kinetics.

114. Foster GD et al. (2003). A randomized trial of a low carbohydrate diet for obesity. New England Journal of Medicine, 348, 2082-2090.

115. Hough, T. (1902). Ergographic studies in muscular soreness. American Journal of Physiology 7, 76-92.

116. Smith, LL (1991). Acute inflammation: the underlying mechanism in delayed onset muscle soreness? Medicine and Science in Sport and Exercise 23,5 543 - 551.

117. Friden J & Lieber RJ (1992). Structural and mechanical basis of exercise- induced muscle injury. Medicine and Science in Sport and Exercise 24,5 521-530.

118. Smith, L et al. (1993). The effects of static and ballistic stretching on delayed onset muscle soreness and creatine kinase. Research Quarterly for Exercise and Sport, 64,1, 103 - 107.

119. Sayers P (1999). The etiology of exercise induced muscle damage. Canadian Journal of Applied Physiology. 24,3,234-248.

120. Peterson J et al. (2003). Ibuprofen and acetaminophen: effect on muscle inflammation after eccentric exercise. Medicine and Science in Sports and Exercise, 35,6, 892-896.

121. Goldfarb AH (1999). Nutritional antioxidants as therapeutic and preventative modalities in exercise induced muscle damage. Canadian Journal of Applied Physiology, 24,3, 249-266.

122. Schwane JA & Armstrong RB (1983). Effects of training on skeletal muscle injury form downhill running in rats. Journal of Applied Physiology 55,3, 969- 975.

123. Myers, J et al. (2002). Exercise capacity and mortality in men referred for exercise testing. New England Journal of Medicine, 346, 11, 793-801.

124. Gulati M et al. (2005). The prognostic value of a nomogram for exercise capacity in women. New England Journal of Medicine, 353,5,468-475.

125. Gulati M et al. (2003). Exercise capacity and risk of death in women. Circulation, 108, 1554-1559. circ.ahajournals.org/cgi/content/full/108/13/1554 (accessed 12/10/07).

126. Drinkwater EJ et al. (2007). Increased number of forced repetitions does not enhance strength development with resistance training. Journal of Strength and Conditioning Research, 21,3, 841-847.

127. Barnett C et al. (1995). Effects of variations of the bench press exercise on EMG activity of five shoulder muscles. Journal of Strength and Conditioning Research, 9(4).

128. Finnie S et al. (2003). Weight lifting belt patterns among a population of health club members. Journal of Strength and Conditioning Research, 17,3,498-502.

129. Welsch E et al. (2005). Electromyographic activity of the pectoralis major and anterior deltoid muscles during three upper body lifts. Journal of Strength and Conditioning Research 19, 2, 449-452.

130. Stoutenberg M et al. (2006). Impact of foot position on electromyographical activity of the superficial quadriceps muscle during leg extension. Journal of Strength and Conditioning Research, 19,4, 931-938.

131. Chandler JT and Stone MH (1991). The squat exercise in athletic conditioning: A position statement and review of the literature. Strength and Conditioning Journal, 13,51-60.

132. Gardner PJ and Cole D (1999). The Stiff Leg Dead Lift. Strength and Conditioning Journal, 21,5,7-14

133. Safran M et al. Instructions for Sports Medicine Patients. Elsevier Publishers.

134. Ross MD (2002). Addressing calf muscle weakness following anterior cruciate ligament reconstruction. Strength and Conditioning Journal, 24,1, 71-72.

135. Antonio J (2000). Nonuniform response of skeletal muscle to heavy resistance training: can bodybuilders induce regional muscle hypertrophy? Journal of Strength and Conditioning Research, 14,1 102-113.

136. Green C M et al. (2007). Effect of grip width on bench press on bench press performance and risk of injury. Strength and Conditioning Journal, 29,5,10-14.

137. Berger A (1991).Effect of tonic neck reflex in the bench press. Journal of Applied Sports Science Research, 5,4,188-191.

138. Levy AM and Fuerst ML (1993). Sports Injury Handbook: Professional Advice for Amateur Athletes. Wiley.

139. Sternlicht E et al. (2007). Electromyographic comparison of stability ball crunch with a traditional crunch. Journal of Strength and Conditioning Research, 21,2,506-509.

140. Crate T (June 1997). Analysis of the lat pull down. Strength and Conditioning, 76.

141. ACSM (1997). ACSM's Exercise Management for Persons with Chronic Diseases and Disabilities. Human Kinetics.

142. Gettman LR et a (1981). Circuit weight training: a critical review of its physiological benefits. The physician and Sports Medicine, 9,44-60

143. Gotshalk, LA et al. (2004). Cardiovascular responses to a high-volume continuous circuit resistance training protocol. Journal of Strength and Conditioning Research, 18,4 760-764.

144. Humburg H et al. (2007). 1 set vs. 3 set resistance training: a crossover study. Journal of Strength and Conditioning Research, 21,2 578-582.

145. Hass CJ et al. (2000). Single vs. multiple sets in long term recreational weightlifters. Medicine and Science in Sports and Exercise, 32,235-242.

146. Calder AW et al. (1994). Comparison of whole and split weight raining routines in young women. Canadian Journal of Applies Physiology, 19,2,185-199.

147. Higbie EJ et al. (1996). Effect of concentric and eccentric training on muscle strength cross sectional area and neural activation. Journal of Applied Physiology, 812173-2181.

148. Keogh J et al. (1999). A cross sectional comparison of different resistance training techniques in the bench press. Journal of Strength and Conditioning Research, 13,3,247-258.

149. Hunter GR et al. (2003). Comparison of metabolic and heart rate responses to super slow vs. traditional resistance training. Journal of Strength and Conditioning Specialists, 17,1,76-81.

150. Keeler LK et al. (2001). Early phase adaptations of training speed vs. superslow resistance training on strength and aerobic capacity in sedentary individuals. Journal of Strength and Conditioning Research, 15, 309-314.

151. Doan BK et al. (2002). Effects of increased eccentric loading on bench press 1RM. Journal of Strength and Conditioning Research, 16,1, 9-13.

152. Brudvig TJ (2007). Identification of the signs and symptoms of acute exertional rhabdomyolysis in athletes: a guide for the practitioner. Strength and Conditioning Journal, 29,1,10-14.

153. Springer BL et al. (2003). Two cases of exertional rhabdomyolysis precipitated by personal trainers. Medicine and Science in sports and exercise,35, 9,1499-1502.

154. Brown B (2004). Exertional Rhabdomyolysis. Physician and Sports Medicine, 34,4.

155. Kao PF et al. (2004). Rectus abdominis rhabdomyolysis after sit ups: unexpected detection by bone scan. British Journal of Sports Medicine, 32,3,253-254.

156. American Heart Association. www.americanheart.org.

157. Wansink B (2006). Mindless Eating.

158. Joubert LM et al. (2006). Exercise, nutrition and homocysteine. International Journal of Sports Medicine and Exercise Metabolism, 16,341-361.

159. Robergs RA & Landwehr R (May 2002). The surprising history of the "HRmax = 220-age" equation. Journal of Exercise Physiology Online, Vol 5, No 2.

160. Bariatric Surgery. In. University of Southern California. Center for colorectal and pelvic floor disorders. www.surgery.usc.edu/divisions/cr/bariatricsurgery.html (accessed 4/8/08).

161. Discovery Health CME: Bariatric Surgery. Weighing the Options. April 7 2007 www.discoveryhealthcme.discovery.com.

162. National Heart, Lung, and Blood Institute, National Institutes of Health (2000). The Practical Guide: Identification, Evaluation, and Treatment of Overweight and Obesity in Adults (NIH Publication No. 00-4084). www.nhlbi.nih.gov/guidelines/obesity/prctgd_c.pdf (accessed 4/7/08).

163. McLean KP et al. (1992). Validity of Futrex-5000 for Body Composition. Medicine and Exercise in Sports and Exercise, 2,.2, 253-257.

164. Seventh report of the Joint National Committee on Prevention, Detection, Evaluation and Treatment of High Blood Pressure. US department of health and human services. www.nhlbi.nih.gov/guidelines/hypertension/jnc7full.htm (accessed 4/17/08).

165. Payne G et al. (1993). Exercise and Vo2max in children: A meta-analysis. Research Quarterly for Exercise and Sport, 64,305-313.

166. Falk B et al. (1996). The effects of resistance and martial arts training in 6-8 year old boys. Pediatric Exercise Science, 8,48-56.

167. Kelly AKW (2005). Practical exercise advice during pregnancy. Physician and Sports Medicine, 33,6. www.physsportsmed.com/issues/2005/0605/weiss.htm (accessed 3/5/08).

168. Sternfeld B et al. (1995). Exercise during pregnancy and pregnancy outcome. Medicine and Science in Sports and Exercise, 27,5,634-640.

169. Clapp JF et al. (1990). Neonatal morphometrics after endurance exercise during pregnancy. American Journal of Obstetrics and Gynecology, 163(6 pt 1):1805-1811.

170. Depken D (1996). Exercise during pregnancy. Concerns for fitness professionals. Strength and Conditioning Journal. October. pp. 43-51.

171. Ireland ML et al. (2000). The effects of pregnancy on the musculoskeletal system. Clinical Orthopedics and Related Research, 372(Mar):169-179.

172. Gerben C (2007). Deep venous thrombosis, upper extremity. E Medicine. ww.emedicine.com/radio/topic774.htm (accessed 3/15/08).

173. Pujol TJ et al. (2007). Resistance training during pregnancy. Strength and Conditioning Journal 29,2, 44-46.

174. Wolf L (1993). In: Skinner JS. Exercise Testing and Exercise Prescription for Special Cases. Lea & Febiger.

175. Gau G. VLDL: What is it? www.mayclinic.com (accessed 5/4/08).

176. Ronai P (2008). Resistance training for persons with osteoarthritis and rheumatoid arthritis. Journal of Strength and Conditioning, 30, 2, 32-34.

177. Ehlke K (2006). Resistance exercise for post myocardial infarction patients: current guidelines and future considerations, Journal of Strength and Conditioning, 28,6, 56-62.

178. Waller, M (2000). Strength and conditioning in multiple sclerosis patients. Strength and Conditioning Journal, 22,2,40-41.

179. No authors. What Causes MS? National Multiple Sclerosis. www.nationalmssociety.org (accessed 5/12/08).

180. No authors. Prednisone. Medline Plus. www.nlm.nih.gov/medlineplus/druginfo/medmaster/a601102.html (accessed 5/12/08).

181. Willardson JM (2008). A brief review: how much rest between sets? Journal of Strength and Conditioning, 30,3, 44-50.

182. Phillips SM et al. (2007). A critical examination of dietary protein requirements, benefits and excess in athletes. International Journal of Sports Nutrition and Exercise Metabolism, 17,S58-S76.

183. Stone M et al. (2006). Stretching: acute and chronic. The potential consequences. Journal of Strength and Conditioning Research, 28,6, 66-74.

184. No authors. Exertional Rhabdomyolysis and Acute Renal Impairment -New York City and Massachusetts, 1988. Morbidity and Mortality Weekly Report. October 26, 1990, 39,42,751-756.

185. Friery, K (2008). Incidence of disease and injury in former athletes: a review. Journal of Exercise Physiology, Online, 11,2, 26-45

Index

hyperlipidemia, 178
hyperplasia, defined, 49
hypertrophy, 49
    training guidelines, 80
hypoglycemia, 181

I

idiopathic hypertension, 176
Initial interview, 11
injury
    ice vs. heat, 171
insulin, 181
insulin resistance, 181
interval training, 87
isometric muscle actions, 53
    functional isometrics, 117
isotonic muscle actions, 53

K

karvonen heart rate formula, 137
    when not to use, 138
ketosis, 181
korotkoff sounds, 161
krebs cycle, 26

L

lactate threshold, 30
lactic acid
    and energy metabolism, 29
    and muscle fatigue, 29
lateral, defined, 32
lats
    inner and outer, 97
leptin, defined, 34
ligaments, 36
low fat foods, 174
lungs, 59

M

macrocycle, defined, 82
macronutrients, 26
manager on duty (MOD), 165
maximum heart rate
    estimating, 135
medial, defined, 32
mesomorph, 153
metabolic equivalents, 140
metabolic syndrome, 181
METs, 140
MI
    defined, 179
mitochondria
    exercise adaptations, 27
mitral valve, 60
motor unit, defined, 44
multiple sclerosis
    exercise guidelines, 186

muscle fiber type
    can exercise change fiber type?, 49
    gender differences, 48
    percentage of, 48
muscle fiber types, 46
muscle mass
    estimating, 158
muscle memory, 54
muscle spindle, defined, 35
muscle tissue
    types, 33
muscular endurance
    and push up test, 146
    and sit up test, 148
    defined, 143
    training guidelines, 79
myofibrils, 42
myoglobin, defined, 46
myosin, defined, 42
myostatin
    and muscle growth, 51

N

near infrared interactance, 158
negatives, defined, 53
nervous system
    central vs. peripheral, 64
    sympathetic vs. parasympathetic, 64
neuromuscular junction, 44
neuropathy, 182
nitric oxide supplements, 62

O

obesity
    and BMI, 152
    and metabolism, 170
    defined, 152
obestity
    and morbid orbesity, 152
OBLA, 30
older adult
    exercise guidelines, 188
organs, defined, 34
osteoarthritis
    defined, 35
osteoblast cells, 39
osteopenia, 185
osteoporosis
    exercise guidelines, 185
overload principle, 72
overtraining syndrome, 159
oxygen debt, 31

P

PAR-Q, 15
percent maximum heart rate formula
    when not to use, 138
percent of maximum heart rate formula, 135
periodization, 81

About Joe Cannon

Joe Cannon, MS, is an exercise physiologist, personal trainer and health educator who resides Pennsylvania. He holds an MS degree in Exercise Science and a BS degree in Chemistry & Biology. He is doubly certified by the National Strength & Conditioning Association (NSCA) as a Certified Strength and Conditioning Specialist (CSCS) and as a Personal Trainer (NSCA-CPT). A dynamic and motivational speaker who specializes presenting accurate information in easy to understand terms, Joe has been a member of the AAAI/ISMA educational facility since 1995, lecturing on the topics of personal training, sports nutrition and dietary supplements. As the Director of Wellness for a health club that ranked among the top 100 of all clubs in the United States, he designed and implemented groundbreaking exercise programs for a diverse range of individuals including seniors as well as those with cancer, osteoporosis, fibromyalgia and developmental disabilities to name a few. Joe has written for several publications including *Today's Dietician, weightwatchers.com, Fitness Management* and the *Journal of Strength and Conditioning.* Joe can be reached directly by visiting his website

www.Joe-Cannon.com

Other Books by Joe Cannon

1. Nutrition Essentials: An information-packed nutrition and sports nutrition textbook that was designed specifically to address the needs and questions of fitness professionals as well as to help them study and prepare for *any* sports nutrition certification. Nutrition Essentials is the companion text to Joe cannon's book on Personal Fitness Training.

2. Nutritional Supplements What Works and Why: A no-nonsense A to Z review of 119 vitamins, minerals, herbs and other supplements. This book cuts through the hype and deciphers what works and what doesn't work, basing all conclusions on scientific facts and rational thought. Over 400 pages in length, this book also highlights side effects that few people in the world have ever heard about. An eye-opening must read for everyone in the fitness industry! Easy to read and highly referenced, this book is the culmination of over 12 years of Joe Cannon's study and investigation of dietary supplements.

3. Personal Fitness Training: The perfect book to help people study and prepare for *any* personal training certification. Joe Cannon reviews not only the essential exercise science topics of personal fitness training, but also how to apply that knowledge to the real world. This book also covers real life issues that fitness professionals encounter each day. Essentially, a college-level textbook that cuts out the technical stuff most trainers don't need while focusing on what they should know, the emphasis of the book is to provide people with the knowledge to work effectively and safely with people and help trainers outshine their competition.

4. Health and Wellness Q & A: This book provides accurate answers to over 135 of the most popular exercise, nutrition and general health questions that fitness professionals are asked every day. Health and Wellness Q & A was created from actual questions fitness trainers and lay persons have asked Joe Cannon over the years. There is no need to search for the answers to peoples questions anymore. They are right here! This is an e-book that can be easily downloaded from Joe Cannon's website.

For more information or to order any of these books visit www.Joe-Cannon.com.

Quick Order Form

To contact Joe Cannon:
      Email: JoeCannonMSCSCS@gmail.com
      Website: www.Joe-Cannon.com
      Mail: P.O. Box 297 Folsom PA 19033

To order a book directly, go to www.Joe-Cannon.com. Notification will be sent when your order is received.

To use this form to order, fill out the entire form and mail to P.O. Box 297 Folsom PA 19033. Notification will be sent when your order is received.

Name:_____

Home Address:_____

City:_____State:_____Zip:_____

Phone number: (_____)_____

Email address _____

Please send me ($25.95) x _____ copies of Personal Fitness Training
Please send me ($24.95) x_____ copies of Nutrition Essentials
Please send me ($24.95) x_____ copies of Nutritional Supplements
Please send me (23.00) x _____copies of Health and Wellness Q & A (e book)
      *Sales tax: Please add 6.00% for all orders shipped to Pennsylvania addresses

Shipping: For orders shipped within the US, please add $5.00 for the first book and $2.00 each additional book. Shipping within the US is free for orders of 10 or more books. For international orders, add $9.00 for the first book and $5.00 for each additional book.

Total book $_____
Sales tax $_____
Shipping $_____
Total $_____

Payment   ´Visa   ´ Master Card   ´ Check

Card number_____

Name on card_____Exp. Date._____

Cardholder's signature_____

I authorize Joe Cannon to charge the above credit card account for merchant services in the amount for products purchased, including appropriate tax and shipping.